An Integrative Approach to Healing Complex and Transgenerational Trauma

This book presents an integrative relational approach to treating trauma and psychological entanglements through autobiographical, philosophical and clinical reflections on the transgenerational dimension of the human experience and the self as an irreducible core of the person.

The book commences with the author's own journey growing up in a Jewish family deeply affected by transgenerational trauma from the Holocaust, providing an inspiring and reflective backdrop to this book's contents. Isaac Pizer then describes and explains his philosophy of therapy, which holds psychotherapy and the treatment of trauma as a relational process that requires an inclusive awareness of the following dimensions of human experiencing: the physical, intrapsychic, relational, transgenerational, transpersonal. Exploring a psychotherapy that holds and integrates transgenerational awareness in the treatment of complex trauma, this book is supplemented with case studies and the author's own experiences.

This compelling and thought-provoking book is intended for therapists, therapists in training and people seeking knowledge and encouragement in their journeys of personal and collective healing, self-realisation and personal growth.

Isaac Pizer is an accredited psychotherapist and a clinical supervisor. Pizer worked for many years as a social worker and commenced training in psychotherapy in 1992. He holds a BSc in Sociology, a Diploma in Gestalt Psychotherapy (2000), an MA in Humanistic Person-Centred Psychotherapy (2003) and a Diploma in Clinical Supervision (2015).

'Reflecting decades of experience as a psychotherapist, this book offers a moving approach to the understanding and treatment of trauma. Isaac Pizer emphasizes an intergenerational framework of understanding and the importance of the human relationship in effecting recovery. Drawing widely from the fields of psychoanalysis, Gestalt therapy, analytical psychology and transpersonal psychology, the text is to be applauded for its scope of reference. With an outlook that is deeply personal without sacrificing its relevance to clinicians, Pizer offers a compelling mediation on Jewishness and the nature of collective trauma'.

Robin S. Brown, *PhD, psychoanalyst in private practice and author of* Groundwork for a Transpersonal Psychoanalysis

'Isaac Pizer re-visions many of the core Gestalt concepts in order to integrate his ideas about trauma and the transpersonal in a way that is a genuine contribution to the Gestalt literature and method'.

Professor Charlotte Sills, *co-author of* Skills in Gestalt Counselling & Psychotherapy, *psychotherapist, supervisor and coach*

'With *An Integrative Approach to Healing Complex and Transgenerational Trauma*, Isaac Pizer has written a wonderfully engaging and soulful account, generously supported with abundant case material and richly substantiated with references from his close acquaintance with the relevant literature, which is a call for us all, in our therapeutic work with psychological trauma, to follow his own journey – as a Gestalt therapist deeply imbued with the radical relationality of Martin Buber – to engage also with the depth of the realms of the transpersonal and the transgenerational. As an integration of theory and practice this book is a veritable tour de force which I found both moving and inspiring, and it will certainly encourage and enrich your own practice as it has mine'.

Dr Gordon Barclay, *MA, MPhil, MRCGP, MRCP, MRCPsych, retired NHS consultant psychiatrist, CAT therapist, founder/trainer of TDS (Towards a Dialectical Self)*

An Integrative Approach to Healing Complex and Transgenerational Trauma

Psychotherapy and the Soul

Isaac Pizer

Routledge
Taylor & Francis Group

LONDON AND NEW YORK

Designed cover image: Getty Images

First published 2025
by Routledge
4 Park Square, Milton Park, Abingdon, Oxon OX14 4RN

and by Routledge
605 Third Avenue, New York, NY 10158

Routledge is an imprint of the Taylor & Francis Group, an informa business

British Library Cataloguing-in-Publication Data
A catalogue record for this book is available from the British Library

ISBN: 978-1-032-59826-0 (hbk)
ISBN: 978-1-032-59823-9 (pbk)
ISBN: 978-1-003-45643-8 (ebk)

DOI: 10.4324/9781003456438

Typeset in Times New Roman
by codeMantra

For my brother Bernard, with gratitude & love,
And all seekers of healing and truth

Contents

Acknowledgements   *x*
Foreword   *xi*

Introduction   1

1 Walking Home   4

2 Transpersonal Theory and the Jewish Contribution to
   Psychotherapy   18

3 My Philosophy of Therapy: The Therapeutic Relationship,
   the Self and Trauma   36

4 Theory and Practice – Relationship, Contact and the
   Healing of Trauma   48

5 Lily, Emily and Angela   67

6 The Transgenerational Dimension   87

7 The Transgenerational Dimension in Practice   97

8 Trauma, Identity Politics and Psychotherapy   113

9 Carrie: Recovery of the Self   128

   Concluding Thoughts   142

Appendix: Clients' Reflections   *143*
Index   *149*

Acknowledgements

I wish to convey my special thanks to Peter Orlandi-Fantini, Grace McDonnell, Charlotte Sills and Elizabeth Pizer for the help and support they have each given me in my long journey of composing and bringing this book to publication.

My heartfelt gratitude and appreciation go to all my clients (whose names have been changed for anonymity) for each gracious permission and contribution.

There are many other people I want to thank for their encouragement, support and help:

Frank R. Bowyer, John Rowan, Anne Johns, Dorle Lommatzsch, Joe Tiernan, Pete Visscher, Sarah Hinds, Peter Baehr, Steve Derrick, Russell Dicks, Susan Kidel, Robin S. Brown, Julie Dearden, Felicia Smith-Kleiner, Nina Will, Niki Reeves, Simon Cavicchia, Carole Turner, Gordon Barclay, Frank Corrigan, Sian Morgan, Reina Lister, Catherine James, Manon Berset, Vinodhini Kumaran, fellow members of the group 'Jewish Relational Psychotherapists', Gottfried Heuer, Susan Kidel, Christopher Eadie, Sandy Marcus, Sandra Maitri and friends in the Ridhwan School UK.

Antonia Salmon is the sculptor who created the candle burner, featured in a poignant moment in Chapter 9. The burnishing tool for the candle burner was created from an ivory-handled hairbrush that originally belonged to her great-grandmother, Ruzena Stutz, who died in Treblinka Concentration Camp. Thank you, Al Skiffington-Smith, for so kindly passing the candle burner into my care.

I want to express my gratitude to all the writers, thinkers and artists whose work has moved, nourished and inspired me. I am especially grateful to Bob Dylan for his indomitable expressions of soul, which sustained me through grim and lonely times.

Foreword

I have just finished reading *An Integrative Approach to Healing Complex & Transgenerational Trauma: Psychotherapy and the Soul* for the second time. It is an understatement to say it is a life's work – it is a life's journey, a book that Isaac Pizer felt it was his duty to write. It contains two major elements: a description of the author's approach to psychotherapy – both in theory and in practice; and also a profound examination of spiritual unfolding. These two elements are inseparable, and this inseparability comes to life in the many rich case studies throughout this book.

This book starts with setting the context: an account of a deeply unhappy boy who carried the legacy of a painful childhood in the North of London, traumatised personally by his own experiences, transgenerationally by persecution of the Jewish people over centuries and intergenerationally through his own family's experience of persecution, dislocation and genocide. It tells of his gradual journey of healing, which he then put to good use in developing his own form of psychospiritual therapy – a transformative blend of Gestalt psychotherapy, psychoanalysis, philosophy, trauma therapies and transpersonal healing. In his own words, it is 'a soulful, relational process for healing and self-realisation'.

This book is indeed an honouring of the 'essential aspect of Self' – the words of A. H. Almaas whom Isaac quotes (among other spiritual teachers) in order to convey his profound understanding of and belief in the spiritual nature of humanity. However, he does not flinch from recognising what is most appalling about humanity – the cruelty, prejudice and oppression that abounds. He looks at it squarely in the face – and yet, he insists on locating it in context of the centrality of the True essential Self. Another quotation from Almaas:

> Essence was there in the beginning, and it is still there. Although it was not seen, not recognized, and was even rejected and hurt in many ways, it is still there. In order to protect itself, it has gone underground, under cover.
>
> (Almaas, 1987, p. 2)

I was intrigued to notice my own reaction as I read all this. Despite being one of the people who tend to focus more on historical and current relational impacts in shaping the self (see *e.g.* Joyce & Sills, 2018), including transferential layers of therapeutic relating (which figure minimally in this book), I found myself moved and persuaded. Isaac offers me a way to bring together what had seemed to be two incompatible parts of me and points to new ways of working therapeutically.

It is important also to stress that this is not only a philosophical and a spiritual work. It is packed with erudition. This book is full of references and quotations, which are not simply acknowledgements, they are treasures. There is a real sense of Isaac appreciatively and powerfully digesting these authors' work in order to learn from them and share their richness with the reader. I feel invited to a gathering, a conference – a confluence of ideas. An example is where Isaac describes the concept of 'self' as it is usually understood in Gestalt therapy theory and extends it thoughtfully and carefully into the spiritual realm. It is not an aggressive elaboration of Gestalt, but an invitation to 'move into the adjacent space', respectfully yet boldly deconstructing authorities such as Perls et al. and Philippson.

Isaac re-visions many of the core Gestalt concepts in order to integrate his ideas about trauma and the transpersonal in a way that is a genuine contribution to the Gestalt literature and method. There is also a wonderful overview of psychoanalytic thought through the lens of Judaic study; an exploration of such trauma concepts as 'Unusual Subjective Experiences' of derealisation and depersonalisation; a deep appreciation of Eastern spiritual knowledge blended with Western psychology; a description of how he uses the Jungian concept of the 'interactive field' as a framework for thinking relationally; an analysis and challenge to the politics of identity and conflict-based responses to trauma…and much more.

I was wondering how I could explain in a Foreword, just why this book is extraordinary. It is not simply that the author shares a moving personal story; nor is it his thoughtful description of his psychotherapeutic approach, nor even the meticulously documented accounts of his clients' lives and therapies. It is something about the love that shines out of every paragraph that makes this book arresting – a love that seems to transcend human frailties and 'entanglements', as he calls them. Rather than attempting to capture what I am trying to say, I invite the reader to start by reading Isaac's Concluding Thoughts at the end of this book. They say it all.

Charlotte Sills
London 2024.

References

Almaas, A.H. (1987) *Diamond Heart Book 1. Elements of the Real in Man.* Boston, MA: Shambhala Pubs Inc.

Joyce, P. & Sills, C. (2018) *Skills in Gestalt*, Fourth edition. London: Sage.

Introduction

This book is for fellow therapists and all who are interested in psychotherapy for complex and transgenerational trauma. It is a personal and professional offering, which I hope will contribute to the compassionate treatment of this deeply debilitating suffering at a time when wars and horrific conflicts span our world, causing traumas which will follow humanity through several generations into the future.

The focus and themes of this book are challenging, and I suggest you allow time to be with and explore the inner experience which arises from reading it. Such a practice can support our personal unfolding and, for those who are therapists, enhance understanding of and empathy with clients. If you are an established or trainee therapist, I hope you find much to draw upon and use in your work with clients. And where you disagree or differ from my perspective, I wish these to be experiences which aid the advancement of your own therapeutic thinking and approach. I consider psychotherapy to be a soulful, relational process for healing and self-realisation. In service to those of us who live with the effects of trauma, I believe in the holding of an inclusive awareness of all the dimensions of human experiencing: the physical, intrapsychic, relational, transpersonal and transgenerational.

With appreciation for Martin Buber's contribution to psychotherapy, I use his concept of relating to another from an 'I-Thou' (1958) attitude as one of reverence for our profound depths, qualities and potential for fulfilment. Trauma is a common aspect of human experience that needs trust, empathy and self-awareness in the quest for its amelioration.

My philosophy and approach contain an explicitly metaphysical, Platonic conception of the self as a fundamental aspect of the person, which psychotherapy can support towards realisation by working through traumas and entanglements that obscure, suppress and thwart it. I consider my perspective concerning the self as being in broad alignment with that of analytical psychology and psychosynthesis, and I value the contemporary contributions of:

- A.H. Almaas, the founder of the Diamond Approach, and his spiritual understanding of the self:

DOI: 10.4324/9781003456438-1

One needs to know the experience of the essential aspect of Self. Self or identity is a specific aspect of Being, a Platonic form, a pure and immutable ontological Presence. When one knows the true Self, the Self of Essence, it becomes possible to see and understand the behavior and attitudes that express it.

(1988, p. 265)

- Robin S. Brown, in his holding of the place and process of the reflective self in psychoanalysis, and in 'Psychoanalysis Beyond the End of Metaphysics: Thinking towards the Post-Relational', offers this important view:

If we set out with an assumption that the individual is merely an expression of the material conditions from which he or she arises, then the patient's experience is inevitably demeaned as a mere epiphenomenon of genetics and/or social conditioning.

(2017, p. 94)

In the first chapter of this book, I share my transgenerational and personal story as a Jewish man born a dozen years after the Holocaust, through which my philosophy of therapy was formed. I commence Chapter 2 by sharing my perspective concerning the transpersonal in psychotherapy, with an outline of transpersonal theories that can complement the therapeutic process. Holding a transpersonal frame, I then look at collective trauma carried through Jewish history, to Sigmund Freud's invention of psychoanalysis, and the remarkable contribution of Jewish men and women to the development of psychotherapy in the twentieth century. It is a story which is encouraging for the therapeutic journey through its exemplifying the fortitude and potential of the human soul (individually and collectively) to transcend suffering with a beneficent answer. This section is also my personal bow to psychotherapy's rich Jewish heritage and a prelude to the philosophy of therapy which I offer in Chapter 3.

In Chapter 4, I explain my thinking and approach to working with trauma. It includes a revision of gestalt therapy for the integration of the transpersonal and transgenerational within the therapeutic frame. Chapter 5 contains three case studies from my work with clients.

I believe transgenerational awareness, the focus of Chapters 6 and 7, is essential for the treatment of complex trauma. Neglecting the transgenerational dimension can cause us to fail to attend to a client and the historical depth of their experience. Such a gap in one's therapeutic consciousness can have the effect of reinforcing intrapsychic suppression and toxic shame experienced by a client. The transgenerational can be the focus or subtlety in the background of work with trauma. An engagement with history passed down *via* entangled relationships and transpersonally can enable an understanding of forms and effects of trauma which have been veiled and hidden. I provide several case studies and vignettes to illustrate my approach and work with trauma, which I hope you will find helpful and encouraging.

Christopher Bollas has written of Europe and America as having 'turned away in significant numbers from introspective living' (2018, pp. 41–42), and this being symptomatic of 'a culture generally uninterested in examination of the internal world, enthralled with the technologies of apps and social networking' (2018, p. xi). With this in mind, Chapter 8 concerns the interface between individual and collective trauma, the politics of identity and the therapeutic process. I argue that whilst awareness of the force and effects of the socio-political dimension upon our lives is important, it is not a substitute for 'introspective living', examining our internal worlds and processing complex and historic traumas. I share personal reflections, along with my analysis and approach as a psychotherapist. The intention behind my disclosures is to offer my personal experience with my thinking and, in this way, not place myself as separate from and above those flaws in the human condition, which recycle and perpetuate the traumas which dominate the human domain.

Now, in the latter stage of my career as a psychotherapist, I see my work has been, in large part, a commitment of service in answer to the horrors of the Holocaust in which people were subject to the most terrible defilement, abuse and murder. Whilst this took place before my birth, it has influenced the way of my soul and purpose in life. In my work with Carrie, there is the presence, connection and interaction of our respective histories. Her therapeutic journey, described in Chapter 9, holds this book's key themes and message concerning the fundamentally irreducible nature and resilience of the self and our potential to heal from complex and transgenerational trauma.

Beneath necessary complexity, the treatment of trauma involves human meeting for the healing of history. In his book, *The Mystery of Human Relationship: Alchemy and the Transformation of the Self* (1998), Nathan Schwartz-Salant writes about the holding of an 'alchemical attitude' in the analytical process (p. 17). We need such trust and commitment, along with humility, knowing that 'conceptual language is inadequate to encapsulate the language of the soul' ('Lament of the Dead: Psychology after Jung's Red Book', Shamdasani & Hillman, 2013, p. 193).

References

Almaas, A.H. (1988) *The Pearl Beyond Price. Integration of Personality into Being: An Object Relations Approach.* Boston, MA: Shambhala.

Bollas, C. (2018) *Meaning and Melancholia: Life in the Age of Bewilderment.* Abingdon, Oxon: Routledge.

Brown, R.S. (2017) *Psychoanalysis Beyond the End of Metaphysics: Thinking towards the Post-Relational.* London & New York: Routledge.

Buber, M. (1958) *I and Thou*, Second Edition. Edinburgh: T&T Clark.

Hillman, J. & Shamdasani, S. (2013) *Lament of the Dead: Psychology after Jung's Red Book.* New York: Norton.

Schwartz-Salant, N. (1998) *The Mystery of Human Relationship: Alchemy and the Transformation of the Self: Alchemy and the Transformation of the Self.* East Sussex: Routledge.

Chapter 1

Walking Home

My philosophy and perspective as a psychotherapist unfolded through the legacy of my family history and the course of the first three decades of my life. I will share this background with you as a prelude to the chapters which follow.

The Background

As a consequence of the Spanish Inquisition of the late fifteenth century, Sephardic Jews settled in large numbers in the Greek city port of Salonika. Their language was Ladino, a hybrid of Hebrew and Spanish. At the beginning of the Second World War, the Jewish population of Salonika numbered more than 50,000 people, but 'during the German occupation almost the entire community 96 per cent of the Jewish population [were]...deported and killed' (Lewkowicz, 2006, p. xvii); with the result that in 1945 'The number of Jews who were registered in Salonika...was 1,950' (Lewkowicz, 2006, p. 69).

My mother, her parents and her siblings, members of the Jewish community of Salonika, emigrated from there to the UK in the early 1930s. Only two of the family members who remained in Salonika survived. Benico Abastado, a first cousin to my mother, survived Auschwitz-Birkenau to settle and raise a family in Israel. The decimation of the family and the tragedy of the Holocaust deeply traumatised my mother, profoundly affecting her way of being as a person and a parent, which inescapably created what I experienced as a pervasive sense of anxiety and tension in our home. Bako and Zana have termed such phenomena as constituting a 'Transgenerational Atmosphere' (2020), and it is explored and discussed in Chapter 6.

I commenced therapy in 1979, but it wasn't until I trained as a gestalt psychotherapist in the 1990s that the psychological significance of my family and community history fully entered my consciousness. With the support of my therapist, course teachers and peers, I became able to face this legacy and was powerfully drawn to visiting Salonika.

2001: A Visit to Salonika

When planning my trip, I decided, despite my limited finances, to book a luxurious hotel in the centre of Salonika, the city that is now called Thessaloniki. I thought

DOI: 10.4324/9781003456438-2

that I would need such comfort amidst the inevitably challenging experiences of the visit.

As my aeroplane began its night descent to Thessaloniki Airport, seeing the lights of the city I was deeply affected by the sense of this visit being a personal pilgrimage. I thought of my loving and inspiring grandfather, Isaac Massarano, and all the previous generations to whom Salonika had been home before the Holocaust.

During my stay in Thessaloniki, there were several occurrences which, in the years since, I have come to accept as fitting into a pattern of serendipity and synchronicity with respect to my relationship with the family's history and the Holocaust.

On the first morning, at breakfast in the hotel, I was surprised and delighted to hear Bob Dylan's 'Mr Tambourine Man' played as background music. Later in this chapter, I write about the significance of this fellow Jew's work in my traversing and surviving adolescence and early adulthood.

In orienting to the hotel's location, surroundings and amenities, I discovered that the Jewish Museum of Thessaloniki was across the road. I entered, introducing myself and seeking information to assist my explorations, and learned that the museum had opened just that week. A formal ceremony to be attended by the Greek Minister of Culture, Chief Rabbi and an Archbishop of the Greek Orthodox Church was scheduled for that Friday, to which I was invited.

I was told that within the now tiny Jewish population of the city, there were still people with the name of Massarano. I was given directions to the cemetery, where people with that name were buried and advised of the train station from which the Jewish community was transported to its fate at Auschwitz-Birkenau. On my visit to the cemetery, I was led by a kindly groundsman to the graves of people with the name of Massarano. I noticed their dates of burial were in the year 1943.

Over the years, an uncle, Michael Molho, had spoken of the Molho bookstore in Salonika. Although there was not a direct family connection, its significance had been impressed upon me. Again, remarkably, I found the bookstore to be a few doors down from my hotel. On entering, I explained the nature of my visit and met Rene Molho, the owner of the bookstore. She was pleased to learn that I had relatives with the name of Molho living in London. Rene selected a beautiful book about the history of the Jews in Salonika for me, of which she had been involved in the production.[1] The bookstore closed a few years later, but an acclaimed film was made about it, narrating the history of the Jewish community of Salonika, Solomon and Rene Molho's survival of the Holocaust, and the restoration and post-war blossoming of the Molho bookstore.[2]

Walking the streets of Thessaloniki, wondering, imagining and gazing at people going about their day, I felt the depth of my family history. I needed to visit Salonika's old train station from which the Jewish community had been transported to Auschwitz-Birkenau. Asking directions from a young woman at the hotel desk, I received a vague answer, which included a question that compounded my sense of darkness and tumult: 'Are Jews connected to the number 666?' I felt disturbed, offended and a little vulnerable, and from these feelings, I responded defensively with a superior tone, tersely suggesting she walk a few doors down and discuss this idea with Mrs Molho.

My search for the train station was difficult. I was lost in a shantytown with dogs running loose. I was anxious, tense and starting to feel overwhelmed when I saw a single-platform station gleaming with a new coat of paint. With the significance of this moment, I moved past the spell of my angst and looked down the track with solemn reverence for my ancestors and their fate.

2014 and 2015: Spiritual Retreats at Auschwitz

In the years that followed my journey to Salonika, I continued to seek therapy for my transgenerational trauma. Family constellation workshops were particularly beneficial to me. I subsequently trained in that modality, which is explored and discussed in Chapter 6.

Seeking spiritual support and nurturing, I also became a student in the Ridhwan School of the 'The Diamond Approach to Personal Realisation', which is a synthesis of Eastern spiritual teaching and Western psychology. It holds an understanding that 'there is a true and timeless Self, an Essential Self, a Self that is not constructed in early life' (Almaas, 1988, p. 265). I have held this belief since a revelatory experience shortly after first commencing therapy (of which I write later in this chapter), from which I began to learn of our potential to heal from trauma and meet each other as 'Thou' (Buber, 1958).

When I learned that fellow students of the Ridhwan School were organising a spiritual retreat at Auschwitz, I saw this as an opportunity for exploration and healing with personal contact and the support of peers, through which I could enable further exploration and processing of the transgenerational trauma and grief which I carry. Looking back, I appreciate how my two retreats at Auschwitz enriched and supported my unfolding as a psychotherapist.

I share below an abridged copy of my article 'My Retreats at Auschwitz 2014 and 2015: Towards Becoming Free of the Past' published in the journal 'Psychotherapy and Politics International' in February 2017. It is reproduced here under license from John Wiley and Sons Ltd. I have provided notes at the end of this chapter to elucidate and reference issues from the article which are explored later in the book.

Retreat May 2014

We stayed at the Centre for Dialogue & Prayer in Oswiecim where we had our early morning and evening sessions. The first day we toured the museum at Auschwitz One. The following four mornings we walked to Auschwitz-Birkenau, the extermination camp. There we had the use of a hut which was used by the SS for recreation; a poignant and darkly transcendent twist of fate. The following few lines came to me shortly afterwards:

Sitting in that hut used by the SS for recreation, and sharing from the depths of our souls. Inquiring, meditating, reciting names of murdered people, reciting

Kaddish, singing, laughing and crying. And seeing a watchtower through the window. This is a metaphor for the journey to freedom which I will hold for the rest of my life.

I experienced deep healing from my contact and companionship with German people on the retreat. Prior to the start of our first walk to Auschwitz-Birkenau, it was suggested we form groups of three. I introduced myself to a German couple. The woman, Monika, reacted with humble distress, upon my informing her of my background: "Is it ok that we walk with you?" I replied from deep within my soul, "It is perfect" – and so it was.

Later in the SS hut, I shared an exercise of personal inquiry with her husband, Volker, in which we each took 15 minutes to speak directly from our feelings and thoughts, whilst the other was a silent witness. Whilst simultaneously viewing one of the camp watchtowers through a window, I looked at Volker, and sensed the different relationship we would have had in this place 70 years ago. Through his writing and a subsequent meeting, I learned that Volker's father was a member of the Waffen SS and worked in concentration camps. In a childhood surrounded by Nazi family and teachers, he had been deeply inculcated with this ideology. I sensed the loneliness and courage of his journey towards spiritual freedom. In the depth and mutual compassion of our second encounter, as I looked at the sensitive lines of his face, I felt our shared kinship.

I was surprised by my experience in walking to Auschwitz-Birkenau each day: on approaching the campus I felt peace, and a powerful sense of connection. The green of the site touched and soothed my open heart. The reciting of the names of family members murdered there, or on route, was cathartic and healing.

Father Manfred, the priest at the Centre for Dialogue and Prayer, told us during the final evening of our stay: 'When you visit you learn that evil is not the last word from Auschwitz, you can sense the spirits want peace'. I was moved by this message, confirming that my experience was neither aberrant nor unique.

On the final morning I walked to the Camp early, the gates opening as I approached. Separating from our small group, alone, in the quiet dewy morning, I found myself bowing with respect, as I walked and explored. Being in solitude in the barracks, sites of the most terrible brutality and suffering, was an especially humbling experience. I kneeled and bowed at a gravestone where ashes were buried and at Crematorium IV, the site of the rebellion of September 1944.[3]

Retreat May 2015

Following my first retreat and visit to Auschwitz, I had monthly Skype meetings with Dorle. She was the instigator and a key organiser of that event. She is a German woman in her early sixties, who has lived in Holland since her late teens. Dorle is a therapist, trainer and teacher of mindfulness.

Whilst there is no evidence or information of Dorle's family being involved in the Holocaust, she has carried a heavy burden of a transgenerational, collective shame and guilt. As a child and young woman, she was deeply disturbed by the post-war atmosphere of her mother country; the hiding from and refusal to speak of awful truths. It was this which compelled her to move to Holland. My attitude during the approaching months to the retreat with Dorle was of heartfelt anticipation and a sense of deep connection. This contrasted with the volcanic grief and tension I experienced prior to the retreat of 2014.

My meeting with Dorle at Katowice airport for our shared journey and exploration at Auschwitz, was for me transcendently significant. With the backdrop of history, it felt like a miracle. Over the year of our meeting and inquiring together, I had come to appreciate Dorle's love and spiritual optimism. My journey back to Auschwitz with Dorle, was an important [healing] movement for my soul. Hearing her experience of disturbance, trauma and loneliness in post-Holocaust Germany, and of her journey away and within, I felt close to her; through both the similarities and differences in our stories.

We again stayed in Oswiecim at CDIM, the Centre for Dialogue and Prayer. I was moved, when Father Manfred said at dinner during our stay, in tired reflection about the propensity of large single national groups to visit Auschwitz, "We can't do the healing alone". He spoke of how Auschwitz can be used to reinforce nationalistic dogmas, rather than support healing dialogue and love.[4]

On the first of our two visits to Auschwitz-Birkenau, Dorle and I set off after an early breakfast for our walk to the campus. It was important to be there early, because of the large groups, who fracture the quiet, which I find crucial. From our visits in 2014, the route along roads cutting across the peaceful Polish countryside was familiar to me. Walking with Dorle was a spiritual experience in itself. I liked our shared, quietly intense attitude. As we walked together, to, and along the paths of Auschwitz.

Arriving at 8 am, there was an incident which reminded me of Rupert Sheldrake's concept of morphic resonance regarding the holding of memory within the fields of soul (Sheldrake, 2011). The Polish guard on the gate, signalled to me that I couldn't enter the campus with my small rucksack. Dorle asked him about her very much larger shoulder bag, and he told her that was fine! At Dorle's suggestion, we solved my problem by emptying the few items I had in my rucksack into her bag, and left the former in the care of the manager of the site's bookshop.

I wondered aloud whether this had been a light historic reflection of the contrasting status of Jews and Germans at this place. As we entered, I felt the love and significance of Dorle's carrying of my load. At Crematoria 2 Dorle recited the names of Jews from her area of Berlin who were murdered in the Holocaust; and I laid on the ground and felt healing in my soul. Each time we entered a barracks, I felt compelled to bow and kneel in the dusty doorway. In one of the barracks we sat together at its centre, in the darkness against a wall, and Dorle lit a candle to accompany her continuing recitation of names of Jews from her area of Berlin who had perished in the Holocaust...[and]...At my request, we sat and inquired together at Crematoria IV, site of the rebellion of September 1944.

I experienced remarkable moments of peace and connection as in 2014, but this time they were more substantially in my body. I felt calmer and at times had a sense of radiant white light, especially around my hands. I also noticed my moving in and out of this experience of presence and awareness, into dissociated, displacing rumination and daydreams. Whilst being an inquiring with Dorle in the grounds of Auschwitz, I noticed an inner movement which had manifested during the several family constellations in which I worked on this issue ten and more years earlier: to lay flat on the ground with my ancestors who had perished. In this position, as in the constellation workshops, I felt comfortable and warm. I eventually followed a subsequent movement in my soul; to stir, kneel, bow and return to my feet.

The night prior to my journey to Poland, I had a nightmare involving knives. During the first evening at CDIM, it occurred to me with some shock that perhaps it related to the fact that Jewish women and men from Salonika were subjected to medical abuse at Auschwitz. Whilst knowing the history, I felt compelled to re-check it via the internet, and in doing so I also found testimony indicating genital medical abuse of Salonikan men. I reflected that from the age of nine, I had experienced pains in my penis, for which comprehensive medical tests revealed no organic cause. These eased and receded as following the psychotherapy which I commenced in 1979. During that first night at CDIM I felt the pains again.

So, on the second day, I felt a need to visit or at least see the barracks where Dr Mengele conducted his medical abuse. Dorle and I found the group of barracks within which it was located. I was struck by their nondescript appearance, and whilst unable to identify the exact barrack in question (probably my propensity to avoid reasserting itself), I kneeled and bowed in the long grass. Just as we were talking about Father Manfred's sadness that individual national and ethnic groups visit Auschwitz with their isolating narratives, rather than sharing and dialoguing with others, I noticed an attitude which caused me salutary shame.[5]

As we approached a barracks which held children, I experienced disappointment, and an inner dismissal and discounting of its significance to me, merely because the barracks' information stand referred to its housing of Polish, rather than Jewish children. I felt pain in my heart, and needed to speak of it to Dorle. This was deeply humbling, and a blow against my own self-righteousness. The next morning we parted at Katowice airport, to meet again on Skype a month later. On returning home, I noticed my regression to a level of anxiety I hadn't experienced for a few years.[6]

My Childhood

My parents carried difficult histories. In their coming together, a veneer of order was formed beneath which was insecurity and incipient chaos. They were people with tumultuous family histories which had spanned the continent of Europe.

My mother lost her keen religious faith because of the Holocaust, and my father had been an atheist since his youth. As a result, the only contact I had with Judaism was through my attendance of the bar mitzvahs of my cousins. My parents were active members of the British Humanist Association.

With respect for the privacy of those members who are alive, my writing concentrates upon my personal experience within this traumatised family. I have endeavoured to distil and convey the qualities of my background and journey and its contribution to my philosophy of therapy.

During my early childhood, my father was a distant, brooding figure whom I felt shy to approach. I am unable to recall his touch, but one day in my teens, my father voiced a pleased, quiet reflection that he could talk to me about philosophy. A door of relationship opened for me, through which I entered with a yearning hunger; eventually, in later years, I was able to appreciate his sadness and sweet, gentle soul.

In contrast to my mother, my father had a quite scant knowledge of his family history, but he would tell me of a great uncle with the same name as him, who was the first person arrested for the East End 'Jack the Ripper' murders, amidst libellous antisemitic newspaper reports and a hateful community frenzy. John Pizer was exonerated to later receive some compensation for the press coverage. He was a member of our family who arrived in the UK during the middle of the nineteenth century, in that large movement of people caused by the anti-Jewish pogroms taking place in Europe.

During the 1940s, my father had been a member of the Socialist Party of Great Britain. Along with several comrades, he came into contact with the philosopher Harold Walsby. They left the Party for a philosophical meeting group led by Walsby and, in its later incarnation, by others to explore and discuss his work. A prominent member of this group was the psychotherapist John Rowan, whom I met in my twenties at these meetings, and significantly for my personal growth in a chance encounter at a café, following which he posted to me an early draft of him, text concerning subpersonalities (Rowan, 1990). I refer to his work in subsequent chapters.

Early memories of my mother contain images of a frightening, shaking, red figure, from which I feel myself tense. She was, in turn, loving, attentive, distant and terrifying; her large shape and loud, cutting voice impacted me from the bedroom door as I lay in the darkness. I found the way to feel close to her was by being a 'good boy'. Her, at times, crazy, annihilating temper caused me to freeze.

My mother knew tragedy on a personal and historical scale. It was present in her eyes and seared through the middle of her voice. She lived on the razor's edge of catastrophe. Her experience and perception of the world were polarised and fearful because of her childhood in Greece, being an immigrant Jew in London, the experience of the Blitz, and the terrible fate of the family that stayed in Salonika.

She was proud of her heritage. Although she lost her religious faith because of the Holocaust, beneath the anxiety, rage and grief which seeped and exploded from her, I feel she never let go of her connection with the spiritual realm. I am grateful for the resonance from that remnant that survived apocalypse and which she conveyed to me.

My mother told me of hunger and the summer heat of Salonika. And her fear, as when the Greek Orthodox Church made processions with incense through the community's streets. I was impacted as a young child by her use of the words 'Germans' and 'Exterminated', as in the ending of stories she told about her beloved Uncle Mentash.

She carried the irreparable distress from a prescient, unbearable vision. Leaving by boat for England with her mother, two sisters and brother, she watched her huddled family waving from the harbour. She saw them small and isolated, wreathed by a halo. Inconsolable, she knew they would never embrace or meet again. I believe my mother's feelings of grief, fear, guilt, rage and desolation expressed the profound suffering of the family's soul. As are the stomach-wracking emotions with which I have lived.

My grandfather, a trader and repairer of fine rugs and needlework, had been earning money for the family away from depression-impoverished Greece, staying in and enjoying the Jewish quarter of Paris. Fatefully, he chose London as the family's ultimate destination.

My mother was a firewatcher during the London blitz and worked in an aircraft factory, where fellow workers told her: 'Hitler's doing a good job with the Jews'... adding as if it could soften the message, 'but you are different', to which my mother would reply: '**No**, I am *very* Jewish'.

Growing up in our household, I developed the habit of ruminating, worrying and daydreaming, which filled the space of my isolation and encompassing fears. I would lie underneath a skylight and enjoy the warm colours which formed behind my eyes.

One day, I asked my mum, 'What is happiness...is it a golden feeling?' Her voice, faint and drifting away, answered, 'I don't know'.

When I was six, my brother came home excited with a copy of the Beatles' record 'Please, Please, Me'. A light had been brought into our home, and receiving their subsequent releases became a personal ritual. Placing a new disc on the turntable, I was excited as I watched it begin to spin, waiting to be touched and enlivened by the warmth and love in their voices. And I felt happy. Each song was like a message from friends, entering me as a fresh charge of spirit and life. In the basement of the shop was a toilet with a skylight and echo. Sitting there, I sang my heart out through their songs, hoping they would hear me, walk into our shop and become my friend.

My physical posture from primary school onwards was hunched and stooped.

I was feeble. Without the skills or confidence to defend myself, I was bullied and attacked by other boys and filled with trepidation on my lone walks home. My mother asked my father to help me with this problem, and he demonstrated a pair of defensive stances: the first, an arm to guard against blows, and the second, his head bowed and shielded by crossed arms. These expressed his perspective regarding the world and his place in it. He did not appear to have confidence in himself or me to assert our right to protect ourselves and be here.

I believe my parents' attitudes and behaviours were symptomatic and expressive of the legacy of many centuries of antisemitic oppression, persecution and genocide. From early in my life, I felt the world to be hostile and dangerous and lived with anxiety and terror. Through therapy, self-reflection and my training as a psychotherapist, I learned that these feelings were manifestations of imprints from a history which included the apocalypse a little more than a dozen years before I was born. My journey of healing led to my study and work concerning the phenomenon and treatment of transgenerational trauma at the centre of this book.

A benefit born of the challenges of my early life was the development of an ability to endure painful emotions. It enables me to be with clients in their suffering and hold empathy and trust in them and their healing. During my training as a practitioner in family constellation work, Judith Hemming offered me a fitting affirmation: 'It was not all in vain'.

Because of my mother's devastating experiences of antisemitism, rather than following Jewish tradition and naming me 'Isaac' after my grandfather, thus identifying me as Jewish at school, she instead gave me the less obvious forename 'Irvin'. Unfortunately, sacrificing the name I was due didn't protect me against the virulent antisemitism which confronted me between the ages of 11 and 16. I had to conceal my Jewishness and contract inside myself. One episode stands out for me:

It was well known that at lunchtime, gangs of boys would walk a quarter of a mile to a Jewish school to 'beat up the Jews'. When I was 13, religious education classes were provided by a teacher who had long hair, dressed in the hippy garb of the time and spoke in a radical and engaging way. One day, he dedicated a lesson to describing the cruelty he claimed was inflicted upon animals by Jewish koshering practices. By the end of the class, a group was shouting, 'Let's go and beat up the Jews'. As we trailed out of the classroom, I looked back at the teacher, sitting silently at his desk with the appearance of a sage. The boys asked me if I would be coming along. I, small and frightened, quietly excused myself from the group and slipped away to disappear for my lonely walk home, where the Holocaust was omnipresent in the atmosphere and behind my mother's eyes.

I was about 11 when my mother shrank and faded into a clinical depression. I remember feeling lost and bereft at seeing her so thin, with the light gone from her eyes. A particularly sorrowful memory is of my finding her scrubbing the living room floor at six in the morning. She spoke to me on her knees, conveying her lostness and desperation, trying to hold on to herself. Mum was admitted to a psychiatric hospital and treated with electroconvulsive therapy. When I was 15, I returned home from school to be greeted by my father informing me that she had attempted suicide by taking tablets and, in parallel with the fate of family members who were murdered at Auschwitz-Birkenau, placing her head in the gas oven. Fortunately, following a short hospital stay, she was able to return home.

I was the second born of my family and drawn into the role of my mother's confidant and counsellor. Through explorations in therapy and family constellation work, I came to understand her expectations of me to be the result of an intergenerational entanglement, for as the second born in the Massarano family, she was assigned the role of carer, whilst her elder sister was idealised and treated differently. It was my mum who was called back from the Land Army to nurse their dying mother, who passed away soon after the end of the War.

My parents' valuing of analytical thought encouraged me to develop my intellect, and my ability to think was a crucial resource and refuge for me. Aligning with their radical political philosophies, I sought meaning and hope through studying sociology and politics. In my mid-teens, I found a small book, a collection of talks from a conference titled: 'The Dialectics of Liberation' (Cooper, 1968). The first chapter is the transcript of the contribution by the radical psychiatrist Ronald Laing, called 'The Obvious'. I took refuge in its critique of the medical model of the mind, with its narrow conception of 'mental illness' through which understanding of the needs and suffering of my family system and its members was being neglected and compounded. The piece, with another by Laing and Esterson (*Sanity, Madness and the Family*, 1970), emphasised what could happen if distress overwhelmed me and broke through into my behaviour. I felt a pressing need to hold onto myself and my thinking.

Bob Dylan was my first spiritual teacher. In the psychologically most perilous years of my life, I was held and sustained by the power of his personal expression and the feeling of connection. His ancestors were part of that great movement of Jews who sought refuge in America from the pogroms of northern and eastern Europe. In his songs, there is, as a figure or background, the theme of isolation and fortitude within a hostile, murderous world.[7] That was the reality for our ancestors, which I have carried as transgenerational trauma.

The perspective in Bob Dylan's songs affected an amplification of my feelings from the family's 'transgenerational atmosphere' (Bako & Zana, 2020) and the projection of my terror onto the contemporary world. I would sit and walk my days, thinking, desperately trying to solve the question: what needs to happen within the human condition for true socialism to be possible? This was symptomatic of my desperate young hope for a world in which I could feel safe.

Being socially paralysed by feelings of fear and shame, I was seeking a sense of potency and hope through my intellect, but inner and deeper dimensions were still largely closed to me. Eventually, the inadequacy of my intellectual pursuit of meaning and peace took me to a dead-end. My ability to sit and study began to evaporate amidst intense somatic discomfort in my chest and genitals. I had been working on an MPhil, and those physical sensations forced me away from studying to gaze out the window.

I sought help.

A Damascene Moment

My damascene moment came a couple of months after commencing my first sessions of psychotherapy with Frank Bowyer, whose approach was a synthesis of gestalt therapy and esoteric teachings.

One night, lying in bed and feeling fear and hopelessness within a thick darkness, I experienced a spontaneous visualisation of my 'inner theatre' to which

Frank had introduced me. A figure like Peter Pan came shooting across the black sky of my inner vision to dive and enter me through the top of my head. I felt instantly transformed, illuminated in my body and soul, with wonder, excitement and hope replacing a void of lostness and fear. I got to know myself and the world anew in the following hours, days and months. I had a vivid sense of self for the first time in my conscious memory, a feeling of being unmistakably me. I felt connected and alive after a childhood and adolescence of frightened and shrunken living.

Since that experience, I have travelled through decades of therapy, exploration and study, guided by a trust in the depth within and between us. As I will describe in Chapter 3, this conviction is central to my philosophy of therapy. I believe that healing and self-realisation happen through deep contact from within and without, transcending limiting normative conceptions of reality. I will share with you a synchronistic experience from my work as a psychotherapist:

In my therapy room, I have a framed photograph of my maternal family from the first decade of the twentieth century (please see Photo 1). One day, during an intense moment of reflection, my client, Robert, looked up at the picture and

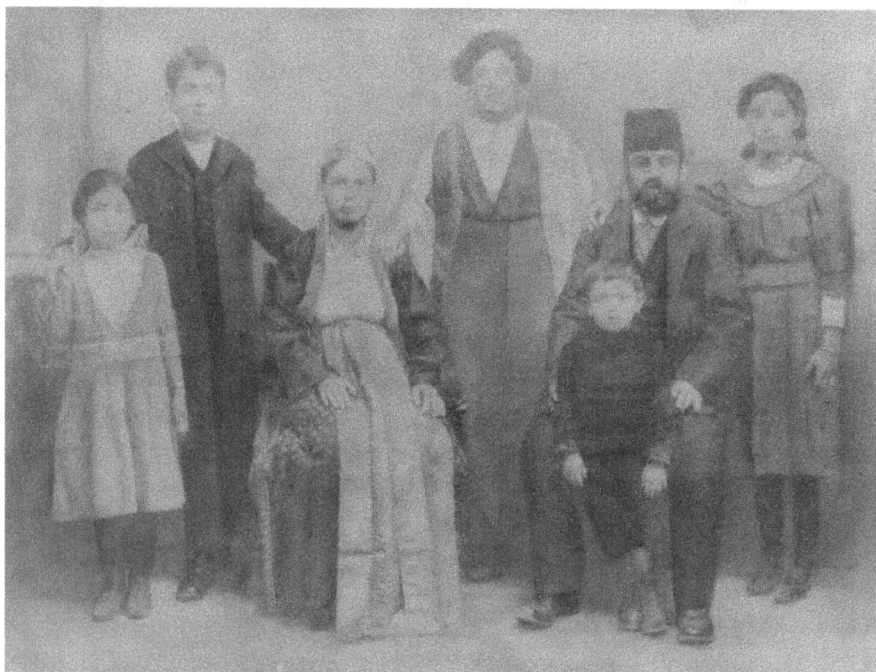

Figure 1.1 Photo 1. My maternal family, Salonika, circa 1908. Polly Massarano is standing first left, my grandfather Isaac Massarano is standing second left, and Luna Massarano in the centre. My great-grandparents, Daniel and Julie Massarano, are seated at the front. Daniel, Julie and Luna perished in the Holocaust.

said 'Family'. A few moments later, it fell, its glass shattering on impact with the floor. My client, in anguish, moved down onto his knees, and I joined him in picking up the pieces for both of our shattered families. Robert's clear, touching account and reflections on this event are included in the appendix, Clients' Reflections.

I hold grief and the most profound respect for those in my community who perished in the Holocaust and the souls who were not allowed to be conceived and born. These lines of a Jewish prayer concisely convey my feelings:

> We mourn for all that died with them; their goodness and their wisdom, which could have saved the world and healed so many wounds. We mourn for the

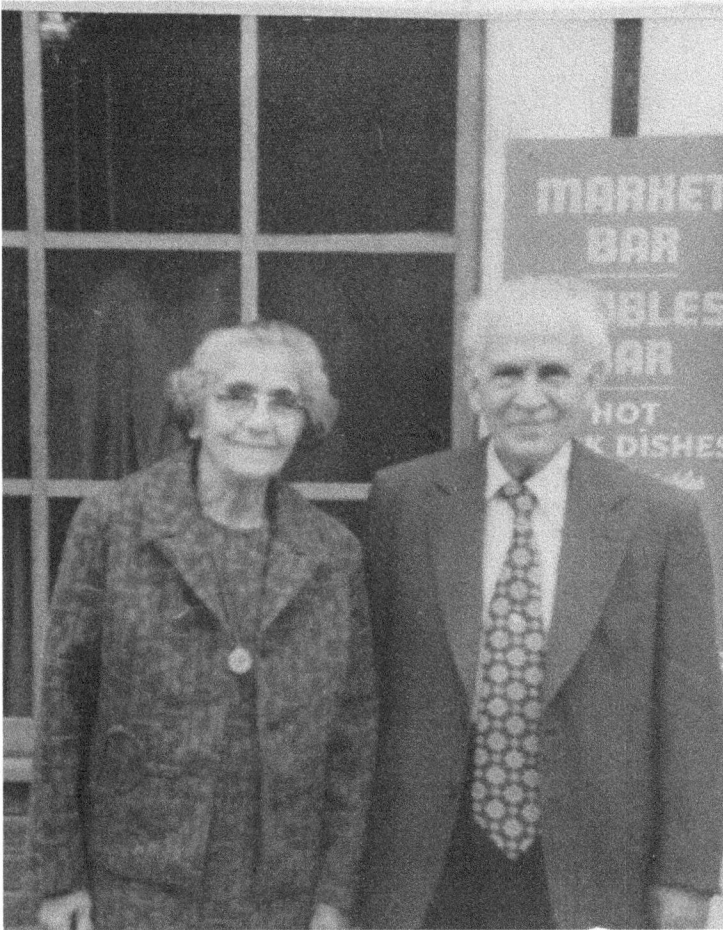

Figure 1.2 Photo 2. Family Renewal. A happy occasion: my grandfather, Isaac Massarano and his Sister Polly Massarano attend a family bar mitzvah in 1975.

genius and the wit which died, the learning and laughter that were lost, and our hearts grow cold as we think of the splendour that might have been.

(Blue & Magonet, 1993)

So, with reverence for my ancestors and their fates, I strive to honour the precious opportunity accorded to me to affirm through my work, the depth and sacred nature of human-being and to help people towards fulfilment in their lives. I believe psychotherapy's central function is to provide healing and support for our opening to inherent, immanent qualities of presence and being. It involves clinical work with the personal, transpersonal and transgenerational dimensions. I have described how these were brought to my awareness through my formative years, and the rest of this book is devoted to the philosophy, theory and practice of a psychotherapy and treatment of trauma which holds them all.

Notes

1 Megas, Y. (1993). 'Souvenir, Images of the Jewish Community, Salonika 1897–1917'. Athens: Kapon Editions.
2 Here is a link to a film about the Molho Bookstore: Els, W. (2013). 'Molho: A Bookstore in Six Chapters'. https://youtu.be/5vFlvQpwn3Y (Accessed: 25 August 2024).
3 In which I understood many Salonikan Jews were involved.
4 In alignment with Father Manfred's insight and my healing and enlightening experience of contact with German people, in Chapter 8 I explore my analysis and concerns regarding the politics of identity and conflict-based responses to trauma.
5 Humbling learning of my own potential for prejudice and indulgence in the politics of identity.
6 Following my return home, I noticed a temporary regression to an intensity of free-flowing anxiety, which I hadn't experienced for a few years. In our first sharing following the retreat, I learned of Dorle's similar reaction. This reminded me of the mystery of the interactive field of the soul and its significance for the practice of psychotherapy, which I write about in the following chapters in this book.
7 There are numerous examples of Bob Dylan's songs with this perspective, and there is a considerable body of academic study concerning his work, such as Wilentz, S. (2011). 'Bob Dylan in America'. London: Vintage Books; Thomas, R.F. (2017). 'Why Dylan Matters'. London: William Collins; and Lathan, S. (Editor, 2021). 'The World of Bob Dylan'. London: Cambridge University Press.

References

Almaas, A.H. (1988) *The Pearl Beyond Price. Integration of Personality into Being: An Object Relations Approach.* Boston, MA: Shambhala.

Bako, T. & Zana, K. (2020) *Transgenerational Trauma and Therapy: The Transgenerational Atmosphere.* Abingdon, Oxon: Routledge.

Blue, L. & Magonet, J. (1993) *The Little Blue Book of Prayer.* London: Fount.

Buber, M. (1958) *I and Thou,* Second Edition. Edinburgh: T&T Clark.

Cooper, D. (Editor). (1968). The Dialectics of Liberation. London: Pelican.

Laing, R.D. & Esterson, A. (1973) *Sanity, Madness and the Family: Families of Schizophrenics.* London: Penguin.

Laing, R.D. (1968) The obvious. In *The Dialectics of Liberation* (pp. 13–33). Cooper, D. (Editor). London: Penguin.

Lewkowicz, B. (2006) *The Jewish Community of Salonika: History, Memory, Identity.* London & Portland: Vallentine Mitchell.

Rowan, J. (1990) *Subpersonalities: The People Inside Us.* Hove & New York: Routledge.

Sheldrake, R. (2011) *The Presence of the Past: Morphic Resonance and the Habits of Nature*, Second Edition. London: Icon Books Ltd.

Chapter 2

Transpersonal Theory and the Jewish Contribution to Psychotherapy

Introduction

In Chapter 1, I shared my personal background and the experiences which led to my commitment to the study and practice of psychotherapy. These included the transpersonal; as transgenerational trauma, synchronistic occurrences and transformative, imaginal events.

In this chapter, I discuss the transpersonal in relation to my philosophy and approach to psychotherapy and later draw upon the 'participatory' theory of the transpersonal to explore the Jewish journey to the creation of psychoanalysis and its crucial contribution to the establishment of humanistic psychotherapy. For the theory and practice of psychotherapy, it is an inspiring illustration of the resilience and qualities available in our souls, which can resource us in our journeys of psychological healing. It is also my bow to Jewish men and women, an honouring of their significant contribution to psychotherapy, which has been neglected due to the effects of antisemitism.

The Transpersonal

I share John Rowan's view that '…the transpersonal is a dimension of all therapy, which requires attention if the therapist is to deal with the whole person who is present …' (2005, p. 1); and the definition he holds of it as '…action which takes place *through* a person, but which originates in a centre of activity existing beyond the level of personhood' (Rudhyar, quoted by Rowan, 2005, p. 29). This perspective allows understanding of the involvement of the transpersonal whenever we explore those experiences, qualities and potentials of the soul, which lie beyond our ego and personality structure. I use the word 'soul' to refer to a spiritual presence within, between and amongst people, which can relate to but be distinct from worldly conditioning.

The need to be conscious of and appreciate the transpersonal, where it has touched and touches us, is highlighted with respect to transgenerational trauma. For that is a process through which our lives have been affected by events one or more generations before we were born. I explore the relationship between the transpersonal and transgenerational dimensions in Chapter 6.

DOI: 10.4324/9781003456438-3

Transpersonal Theory and Psychotherapy

In the process of psychotherapy, there is a complex, dynamic relationship between personal and transpersonal experiencing. Psychotherapy is a context for exploring and appreciating spiritual emergence and emergency (Grof & Grof, 1989) as non-normative expressions from our depth, which provide us with guidance and nourishment. Furthermore, in the treatment of trauma and clearing of intrapsychic occlusion, psychotherapy can enable our opening to and deepening experience of the transpersonal and spiritual. I will here outline theories concerning the transpersonal, which I have found complementary to my work as a psychotherapist. If you would like to learn more about the history and range of perspectives concerning the transpersonal, *The Wiley Blackwell Handbook of Transpersonal Psychology* (Editors: Friedman & Hartelius, 2015) is an excellent resource book.

The Perennial Philosophy

In the *Underlying Religion: An Introduction to the Perennial Philosophy* (2007), Martin Lings and Clinton Minnaur define the perennial philosophy as: '… both absolute truth and infinite Presence. As absolute Truth it is the perennial wisdom (*sophia perennis*) that stands as the transcendent source of all the intrinsically orthodox religions of humankind' (p. xii).

With its trust in the depth and commonality of the pathways to spiritual realisation, this perspective can be one which sustains people through the challenges of psychological healing and personal unfolding. I believe such trust and concordant humility is expressed by Roberto Assagioli, the founder of Psychosynthesis, when he writes of the transpersonal and the experience:

> …of the enduring, immortal essence of the spiritual "I", the Self…It is here that one comes into contact with Mystery, with supreme Reality. Of this I am unable to speak…However, psychosynthesis can help us to approach it and reach the very threshold.
>
> (1991, p. 31)

The perennial philosophy holds a vision of a 'single spiritual ultimate' (Hartelius & Ferrer, 2015, p. 189), named by Aldous Huxley as 'the universal immanence of the transcendent spiritual ground of all existence' (1945, p. 7). A person's spiritual journey is understood to be towards what Ken Wilber called 'unity consciousness'. Wilber observes:

> …So widespread is this experience of the supreme identity that it has along with the doctrines which purport to explain it, earned the name "The Perennial Philosophy". There is much evidence that this type of experience or knowledge is central to every major religion…so that we justifiably speak of the "the transcendental unity of all religions" and the unanimity of primordial truth.
>
> (2001, p. 3)

It is vital to respect clients where they perceive, experience and express glimmerings from the transpersonal depth. With an attitude similar to Assagioli's, Huxley writes in *The Perennial Philosophy* (1945):

> The divine Ground of all existence is a spiritual Absolute, ineffable in terms of discursive thought, but (in certain circumstances) susceptible of being directly experienced by the human being.
>
> (p. 21)

The perspective of *The Perennial Philosophy* is present in three of the four approaches to which I refer in this chapter, and it can be valuable in psychotherapy for holding and sustaining meaning through the challenges that arise. In my work with Carrie, to which Chapter 9 is dedicated, this was the case with respect to my holding and expression of a soulful, essential trust in her and her journey when she was assailed by despair.

Three Categories of Consciousness and Functioning

The following three categories are helpful for an integrated practice of psychotherapy, which is attentive to our movement between different levels of consciousness and ways of relating to self, the environment and life. With the exception of participatory theory, they are broadly in line with the perspectives of the transpersonal models to which I refer in this chapter:

- **Pre-personal**: Present before the formation of a functioning ego, this is a developmentally primitive consciousness, to which we can regress, for example, as a result of shock and trauma, which cause the impedance or suspension of our capacity to orient. It is manifest in magical thinking (albeit possibly expressive of a connection with the spiritual), where there is an unreflective pursuit of desires and hopes and the absence of a mature consideration of material and environmental conditions.
- **Personal**: This is where we are oriented to the material world and social environment we inhabit, with its configurations of beliefs, norms and values, but are less available to the more expansive experiences of soul and spirit, which are present beyond our egoic consciousness.
- **Transpersonal**: Here, one's process is exemplified by a capacity for free, non-normative and reflective experiencing and relating, including the dimensions of soul, spirit and the ground of being.

Michael Washburn: The Dynamic-Dialectical Model

I find Michael Washburn's approach to the transpersonal (1995) helpful. Influenced by the work of Jung, he provides a theory of human development that incorporates the transpersonal. Washburn describes the individual's early separation from the 'dynamic ground' ('Great Mother') of being in our development of a functioning ego for relating and the satisfaction of needs and egoic desires within the world. He explains how the limitations of and dissatisfaction with egoic life can lead us in adulthood towards a rapprochement with the depth of being held by the dynamic ground, bringing the realisation of a spiritually integrated life. Alongside Jung's concept of individuation, concerning the different stages in a person's life, this model is helpful for the identification and understanding of a client's development through their personal journey. In the case studies of my work with Emily and Lily in Chapter 5, we can see the importance of exploring transpersonal aspects of their experiences through work with dreams and imagination, which took them beyond the restrictions of the ego and personality structure formed during infancy.

Ken Wilber: The Structural Hierarchical Model

Another approach to the transpersonal, which I find useful, is from the work of Ken Wilber. He provides a schema concerning the different levels of consciousness we can inhabit in our lives and through the dialogue and explorations of psychotherapy. It is a conceptual spectrum, with each level constituting a holistic pattern of being and consciousness within a 'nested hierarchy (or holarchy)' (2000, p. 7) concerning our psychological and spiritual functioning. For the practice of psychotherapy, Rowan (2005, pp. 80–81) has provided elucidation of Wilber's model, which can aid understanding of how and what a client might comprehend, experience, need and speak in psychotherapy:

- **Instrumental Self**: *Definition*-I am defined by others; *Motivation*-Need; *Personal Goal*-Adjustment; *Process*-Healing & Ego building
- **Authentic Self**: *Definition*-I define who I am; *Motivation*-Choice; *Personal Goal*-Self-actualisation; *Process*-Ego development
- **Transpersonal Self (Soul)1**: *Definition*-I am defined by the Other(s); *Motivation*-Allowing; *Personal Goal*-Contacting; *Process*-Ego Reduction
- **Transpersonal Self (Spirit)2**: *Definition*-I am not defined; *Motivation*-Surrender; *Personal Goal*-Union; *Process*-Enlightenment

Wilber writes:

> … individual development through the various waves of consciousness is a very fluid and flowing affair. Individuals can be at various waves in different circumstances; aspects of their … consciousness can be at many different waves…
>
> (2000, p. 7)

In my work with Carrie (to whom Chapter 9 is dedicated) and her experience of complex trauma, attention to her movement between different 'waves' of consciousness enhanced my attunement to her needs and process. In this intense dialogic process, it was also important to be attentive to and informed by my shifting consciousness, as our explorations impacted me and my history. I believe this quality of attention is crucial for empathic work, which honours and supports the whole person.

A.H. Almaas: The Diamond Approach

In the course of personal therapy and my training in family constellations work (an important transpersonal model in relation to transgenerational trauma, discussed in Chapter 6), I became acquainted with A.H. Almaas's 'Diamond Approach' and joined his Ridhwan School as a student in 2005. The Ridhwan School's information about its teaching of Almaas's Diamond Approach (https://online.diamondapproach.org/rf-is-aus/) advises that it is neither a psychotherapy nor an approach to healing. However, I have found the Diamond Approach to be a transpersonal and spiritual model which can be complementary to the psychotherapeutic journey. It has enriched my personal life and professional practice.

The Diamond Approach holds both Eastern spiritual knowledge and Western psychology in its teaching and affirmation of the depth and potential of our being, and this attitude is central to the integrative form of psychotherapy I describe in this book. It is present in Almaas's 'The Pearl Beyond Price. Integration of Personality into Being: An Object Relations Approach' where he states:

> An important part of our exploration in this book is to study in detail and in depth the findings of depth psychology…and relate them to the spiritual perspective of the man of spirit.
>
> (1988, p. 10)

The Diamond Approach's integrated conception of human development, of our relationship with 'essence' the ground of being, early developmental alienation from the former, and the transpersonal 'Inner journey home' (2004) has similarities to Washburn's neo-Jungian conception. It affirms and supports our potential for reconnection with essence, towards personal realisation, *via* individual, group and communal exercises of 'inquiry' (2002), and mindfulness and meditation practices.

Almaas articulates an understanding of the role of trauma in our becoming alienated from the ground of being and essence, through which the self goes 'undercover', and our personality develops as the normative, relationally adaptive, protective 'cover' (1987, pp. 1–2). He notes that 'unmetabolized history not only limits one's capacity to traverse the path, but also distorts it and its experiences' and that some of us will require trauma therapy before 'fully engaging' in the spiritual journey (2004, p. 628). With its inclusion of the transpersonal and transgenerational in the exploration of trauma, I believe my approach can be helpful in this respect. I have included vignettes from my work with two students of the Diamond Approach: John in Chapter 4 and Sabine in Chapter 8, whose capacity for psychotherapeutic exploration had been fostered through engagement with the Diamond Approach.

Martin Buber

In Chapter 3, I explore Buber's concept of I-Thou (1958) as an attitude at the heart of my philosophy and approach as a psychotherapist. You will find its presence within this book's vignettes and case studies.

Buber's Jewish and existentialist philosophy is deeply rooted and expressive of Judaic history and places dialogue as central to human existence and contact with the divine. It was further developed for the practice of psychotherapy by Friedman (1985), Hycner (1993) and Hycner and Jacobs (1995), and it has had a very significant influence on humanistic psychotherapy. Buber's is a co-creative, relational perspective concerning human and religious relationships from which insights, understanding and healing arise through contact and dialogue. The engagement with the other as 'Thou' is both a therapeutic and metaphysical stance. It is an attitude of trust in the individual and divine immanence to which I commit myself in my work with clients. The conception drawn from Buber of psychotherapy taking place in the 'between' (Hycner, 1993) of the therapist-client dialogue is an understanding of both therapy and the transpersonal as participatory processes.

Participatory Theory

Jorge Ferrer and Glen Hartelius (2015) argue that there are only two major paradigms of transpersonal theory: The perennial philosophy and 'participatory' theory.

Ferrer is a pioneering author of the latter. He understands the transpersonal as a 'mystery', enacted through a co-created participatory process, for which 'Spiritual cocreation has three interrelated dimensions-intrapersonal, interpersonal and transpersonal' (2017, p. 11).

Participatory theory considers:

> ...transpersonal phenomena as pluralistic events that can occur in multiple loci (e.g., an individual, a relationship, or a collective) and whose epistemic value emerges-not from any preestablished hierarchy of spiritual insights-but from the events' emancipatory and transformative power on self, community and world.
>
> (Ferrer, 2017, p. 9)

In contrast to *The Perennial Philosophy*, participatory theory eschews the conception of a single spiritual ultimate, instead understanding the transpersonal as 'An ocean with many shores' (Ferrer, 2002, p. 144). Ferrer suggests, rather than assessing transpersonal models and traditions according to 'a priori doctrines or a prearranged hierarchy of spiritual insights' (2017, p. 10), that we consider them in relation to their freeing of people from narcissism and self-centredness, supporting personal blossoming and integration, and the fostering of 'ecological balance, social and economic justice, religious and political freedom, class and gender equality and other fundamental human rights' (2017, p. 18).

Transpersonal Theory and the Practice of Psychotherapy

I believe knowledge of the different traditions and theories concerning the transpersonal is important for understanding the range of human experiences and belief systems lived by clients. However, the psychotherapy relationship is not the place to hold and impose determinations concerning philosophical disputes about the nature of the transpersonal, but to be alongside a client in their individual and collective experiencing of it. I view the different models of the transpersonal to which I have referred as each being of potential value in psychotherapy, and agree with Washburn (2003, 2020) that they do not need to be considered in opposition or competition with each other. I also note Ferrer's statement: 'My sense is both the participatory and Wilberian visions can accommodate spiritual diversity in different ways' (2017, p. 204).

I believe a client's journey of healing and unfolding will be supported by our humility and care concerning their personal experiencing. With this attitude, we can help a client's exploration and inquiry into:

- An experience of a religious or spiritual logos characteristic of the tradition of *The Perennial Philosophy*.
- A sense of personal development, for which narratives such as those provided by Wilber, Washburn and Almaas might be helpful.
- Relational, collective and systemic experiences that may be understood through the participatory perspective offered by Ferrer.

Section Two: Psychotherapy and the Jewish Journey

Participatory theory supports understanding of the co-creative capacity of soul and souls for endurance, brilliance and a fulfilment of personal, collective and transpersonal dynamics. This, I believe, was the case with respect to the Judaic journey, which led to the creation of psychoanalysis and the crucial role of Jews in the development of humanistic psychotherapy in the mid-twentieth century. These achievements emerged through Judaic culture and were fruits of the Jewish path through exile, persecution and genocide. To look at such inspiring examples of the process of soul allows support for a soulful-psychotherapeutic perspective, which can encourage us on our respective journeys. This is a story intimate with my heritage and my heart.

The Transpersonal Legacy and Bequest

The Jewish creation of psychoanalysis and immense influence upon the general development of psychotherapy have been and are an extraordinary contribution from a demographically small ethnic group and race of people. I consider it to be a participatory-transpersonal process in the holding and transfiguration of worldly and spiritual experiences.

In the Jewish peoples' traversing of millennia marked by exile and persecution, they related and engaged with God dynamically, transforming their religious, collective and personal experiencing; from which foundations for psychoanalysis and humanistic approaches to psychotherapy were formed. I will outline this historic process, which involved a radical change in religious practice from one led by priests and ceremony to that of ritual and dedication to truth and the divine through the examination, debate and reflection upon sacred texts. In this way, a philosophy, practice and culture of intense hermeneutic work were formed concerning a people's relationship with God, truth and fellow humans.

Brian Lancaster has explored Jewish mysticism in relation to participatory theory (2008), with emphasis upon the Judaic conception of the co-creative relationship between God and humanity that:

> God requires human participation... to promote his own wholeness (p. 174)...
> [and] Human creativity recapitulates divine creation, and the concealed fount
> of our creativity is the meeting ground between the human and divine minds.
>
> (p. 186)

Lancaster concludes his work with the following lines through which we can understand the creation of psychoanalysis and the establishment of humanistic psychotherapy as a manifestation of the participatory-transpersonal:

> ... the vicissitudes of Jewish history, the narrative of exile and redemption is
> powerfully founded in the exigencies of oppression. Yet the genius of the Jew-
> ish mind peered through historical eventualities into the concealed existential
> mirroring of God and man.
>
> (p. 189)

Ambivalence, Avoidance and Antisemitism

Harvey Schwartz, in his preface to 'The Jewish Thought and Psychoanalysis Lectures' (2020), alluding to a background of antisemitism and the benefits of acknowledging and exploring the Jewish contribution to psychoanalysis and psychotherapy, writes:

> ...[an] intention of this lecture series was to make overt what has long been la-
> tent. The historically high percentage of psychoanalysts who have been Jewish
> is both well known and unspoken. ...The purpose of this text... is to bring to
> light that the fears we associate with speaking freely of such matters need not
> limit us. Curiosity, not to mention pride in one's cultural affiliation invites others
> to feel the same about their own heritages.
>
> (p. xiv)

I carried the fear and toxic shame which I described in Chapter 1 into my training as a Gestalt psychotherapist in the early 1990s. In response, I received a compassionate and life-changing tribute to my Jewish heritage from the trainer, Ken Evans. He believed that without the legacy provided by Jewish men and women, his psychotherapy training institute probably wouldn't be in existence. In more than 30 years of attendance at hundreds of professional conferences, workshops and seminars since then, I have not heard another reference to the crucial role of Jews in the development and blossoming of psychotherapy. But, I have listened to claims that Western psychotherapy has been dominated by 'White men'; to which I infer dismissal or ignorance of the Jewish pioneering practitioners and writers (men and women) to whom Ken Evans referred with immense respect. Stephen Frosh, in his book *Hate and the 'Jewish Science' Anti-semitism, Nazism and Psychoanalysis* (2005) notes the Jew as 'The Other' and 'a kind of "universal stranger" for Western society' (p. 198), and it is apposite concerning such pointed or ignorant acts of omission. As is Schwartz's reflection, in discussion of Sigmund Freud's final book 'Moses and Monotheism' that, 'The Hebrew people were not only the "founders" of Western culture…but also "the Other" to the very culture they unwittingly founded' (2020, p. 31).

This is a thesis central to Nirenberg's 'Anti-Judaism: The History of a Way of Thinking' (2013), who concluded that:

> The "Jewish" terrors that assailed Germany and many of its neighbours in the first half of the twentieth century were not reflections of reality, or eccentric fantasies imposed on a populace by a powerful propaganda machine, or even of a profound but demonic possession of the German nation between 1933 and 1945… They were rather the product of a history that had encoded the threat of Judaism into some of the basic concepts of Western thought, regenerating that threat in new forms fitting for new periods, and helping far too many citizens of the twentieth century make sense of their world.
>
> (Nirenberg, 2013, p. 459)

Amidst the intensifying manifestation of antisemitism in late nineteen and early twentieth-century Europe (Klein, 1985), Sigmund Freud was very concerned about the danger it posed to his fledgling psychoanalysis, for the latter to be and dismissed as a 'Jewish science' (Frosh, 2005, pp. 1–2). Thus, he considered it highly significant when Carl Jung joined the circle of psychoanalysts in 1907 who met with him in Vienna, of which the membership had previously comprised solely of Jews. Despite an awareness of Jung's antisemitism, Freud viewed his membership of the group as crucial. Jerry Diller, in 'Freud's Jewish Identity: A Case Study in Ethnicity' (1991), writes that Freud being 'desperate' for 'non-Jewish support' (p. 179), told Karl Abraham: 'Our Aryan colleagues are quite indispensable to us' … 'otherwise psychoanalysis would fall a victim to anti-semitism' (p. 183).

In line with the global nature of antisemitism, Celia Brickman (2010, p. 35) observes and appreciates that the subsequent generations of Jewish psychoanalysts, who fled pogroms and Nazism for the USA, were for the latter to be and assimilation into the host country and tended to distance themselves from and avoid publicising their Jewish identities and religion. Perhaps the humanism of psychoanalysis and its unifying philosophy, which Dennis B. Klein discusses in *Jewish Origins of the Psychoanalytic Movement* (1985, pp. 148–150), may have also discouraged them from drawing attention to their ethnic and religious identity and heritage.

Alongside the reasons provided by Schwartz, it is appropriate to uncover and highlight the contribution of Jews to psychoanalysis and psychotherapy in support of an understanding of participatory-transpersonal processes and an appreciation of the potency and agency of the soul to transcend and transfigure immense suffering and challenge, for healing and the benefit of humanity.

History and Legacy

I believe the Jewish creation of psychoanalysis and immense contribution to psychotherapy more generally needs to be understood in transpersonal as much as intellectual terms, for appreciation of the potential of soul in relationship with the divine (In Judaism: God), to survive, transcend and transform experience. This is a legacy which developed through and was delivered from struggles with adversity, which can inspire and support us, and the process of psychotherapy. It was/ is a participatory-transpersonal phenomenon formed by Judaic culture, beliefs and communal practice.

The Jewish people, through a history in which they suffered expulsion and exile from their homeland, and persecution and genocide in their diaspora across Europe, developed the practice of Judaic scholarship analysis, reflection and debate concerning religious experience, truth and human reality. The latter two are matters at the heart of psychoanalysis and psychotherapy, with religious practice transmuted in dedication towards understanding the unseen, unconscious and mystery in the human experience. This is reflected in these words from Lewis Aron, the relational psychoanalyst, whose work to which we are indebted for an understanding and appreciation of the relationship between Judaism and psychotherapy:

> From the moment that Freud identified interpretation as his method of creating meaning, psychoanalysis became inextricably linked to, and some may say, a continuation of Jewish thought.
>
> (2010, p. 16)

Philip Cushman (2010) describes a development in Judaism, instigated by the Pharisees approximately 2,000 years ago, whereby it began to move away from hierarchy and a concentration upon ceremony and sacrifice at Temple in Jerusalem towards a focus on the divinity of the Word as contained in the Torah (The Hebrew

Bible) and Jewish oral tradition. This was a prudent move because with the Roman destruction of the Second Temple in 70 C.E., Jews were thrown into exile without a central location for the holding of religious practice and experience:

Cushman writes:

> Without the concrete relation embodied in the smoke of the Temple's animal sacrifices, they desperately needed a new way of understanding and then enacting their relation with God. The Pharisees accomplished both through the creation, systematic collection, and arrangement of small, everyday social practices and customs that were necessitated by the ever-new challenges brought on by new historical circumstances in both Judea and the diaspora. They came to warrant, describe and explain their practices and customs through biblical commentary and legal texts (p. 375)...
>
> [With] the Jewish nation's defeat and exile, the rabbis were acutely aware of God's absence in the world.... A limited solution was achieved... through the learned capacity to tolerate absence, through everyday rituals, the beginning of group prayer, and the communal study of the texts.
>
> (p. 377)

Thus, through the Jewish peoples' travails, Judaism developed to manage God's absence and inaction through communal ritual and the practice of Midrash, which is the examination, hermeneutic interpretation and commentary upon holy texts. In this, both devotional and critical orientation towards the Word, mysterious and multi-layered with meaning, 'They found God and a new understanding of God's presence, in the gaps of the text' (p. 384).

In *Repair of the Soul: Metaphors of Transformation in Jewish Mysticism and Psychoanalysis* (2008), Karen Starr explores the relationship between the Kabbalah, the Judaic body of 'creative commentary... mystical reinterpretation of biblical and rabbinic literature' (p. 4), and psychoanalysis, observing:

> The Kabbalah characterizes the journey toward self-understanding and self-realisation as tikkun, or repair, by which the particular spark unique to one's soul is enflamed and restored to its source in the divine, transforming God himself in this process. The endeavour to know the self deeply is conceived as the movement toward God in relationship.
>
> (p. 11)

In Freud's work, there is an intense study and commitment towards the self and 'The Unconscious' (Freud, 2005), which parallels both the analytical culture of Judaism and the fortitude of the Jewish people. Starr discusses Freud's Hassidic background and the relationship of his work to Jewish mysticism (pp. 16–19). She also explores Wilfred Bion's revision of psychoanalysis, which we can consider to be one which is revealing of its Judaic mystical roots. She observes that Bion 'defines the goal of the analytic process in words that could have been spoken by a kabbalist articulating the cosmic processes put into effect by personal transformation...' (p. 40).

Sigmund Freud and His Colleagues

A gift was formed for humanity through the Judaic commitment to and connection with the divine *via* hermeneutic study, analysis and debate and the transmuting of religious practice and experience. It was delivered by an Austrian Jew and his Jewish colleagues. Amidst the antisemitism which foreshadowed the Holocaust, they brought innovative attention and care to psychological suffering, and, as we know, the answer from the world was genocide.

Dennis B. Klein (1985) describes the evaporation of nascent liberalism and intensification of antisemitism in nineteenth-century Europe, in which Jewish hopes and aspirations for assimilation were rebuffed, providing a desperate impetus for Zionism and the eventual establishment of the modern state of Israel, and the creation of psychoanalysis. Concerning the latter, Klein observes: '... the movement and the theory of psychanalysis illuminate the emergence of self-assertion among German Jews, as well as the way this inner transformation impelled Jews toward restoring mankind to the idea of universality' (p. 32); they had 'renounced their assimilationist aspirations and examined the only free realm left to them, the inner life of the psyche' (p. 14). Klein describes, both broadly and with personal detail, the importance of Jewish identity, history and philosophy to Freud and the members of the psychoanalytic community he established. Klein considers this background to argue '...for the interpenetration of the Jewish redemptive vision with the psychoanalytic movement's redemptive hope for the eradication of neurosis' (p. 139).

With such an understanding, we can see how Jewish history, religious practice and culture, with its commitment to God and truth, brought to Europe (in an epoch of both invention and ominously aggressive antisemitism) the creation of psychoanalysis and the transformation of psychotherapy. With a heritage and culture of commitment to 'tikkun', the 'repair of the world' (Starr, 2008), I believe psychoanalysis emerged as an ostensibly secular transfigurative creation out of Jewish suffering, fortitude and dedication. It is concerned with the psyche as towards an absent God, being attentive to the psyche's hidden territory of the unconscious.

Whilst emphatically atheist, Freud's identity, commitment and work were intimately intertwined with Judaism. Stephen Frosh (2005) explores Freud's Jewish identity *via* his correspondence, lectures and writing, with particular reference to his books Totem and Taboo and Moses and Monotheism, to inform the reader of the connection between Freud's Jewish identity and his dedication to the establishment and prospering of psychoanalysis.

Frosh quotes Freud from Moses and Monotheism, where he refers to the establishment of the first Torah school following the destruction of the second Temple: 'From that time on, the Holy Writ and intellectual concern with it were that what held the scattered people together' (2005, p. 32). Frosh follows that quote with another, from Freud's last address to the Vienna Psychoanalytic Society in 1938 following the Anschluss (Nazi Germany's annexing of Austria) and before his escape to London. Again, referring to the establishment of that first Torah school, Freud said:

> We are going to do the same. We are, after all, used to persecution by our history, tradition and some of us by personal experience.
>
> (2005, p. 32, from Diller, 1991, p. 206)

Following that moving proclamation from Freud, Frosh closes in on a significant conclusion:

> Here, the identification between psychoanalysis and Jewish thought is absolutely explicit, as is the psychoanalytic movement and the Jews. It is as if Jewish history has translated directly into psychoanalytic history, the latter being the continuation of the former...
>
> (Frosh, 2005, p. 32)

In those words, we can see the breaking through of a passionate expression of Freud's complex Jewish identity (as explored by Diller, 1991) and his respect for the historic Jewish journey through exile and suffering.

Klein, in emphasising the coupling of Freud's Jewish identity and life's work, reflected:

> Freud aimed at liberating humanity from repression and neurotic misery through an arduously uncompromising commitment to truth...[Otto]Rank saw his Jewishness as a condition of redemption; Freud saw it as a precondition, a preparation for the psychoanalytic task.
>
> (1985, p. xvi)

Freud, despite his atheism and commitment to secular discourse, upon his arrival in England following the last journey of his long life, delivered a stirring declaration and reference to spiritual values for representatives of the Hebrew community of London who greeted him. It is a statement which supports the participatory-transpersonal appreciation of the Jewish journey I am offering:

> We Jews have always known how to respect spiritual values. We preserved our unity through ideas, and because of them we have survived to this day.
>
> (Diller, 1991, p. 122)

And, aligned with this expression of solidarity with and respect for Judaism, in "'I Knew the Method": The Unseen Midrashic Origins of Freud's Psychoanalysis', Jennings and Jennings (1993) provide understanding concerning the relationship between Midrash and Freud's psychoanalytic methodology. Handelman, in *The*

Slayers of Moses: The Emergence of Rabbinic Interpretation in Modern Literary Theory (1982), stated this view most emphatically:

> Freud absorbed the Midrashic hermeneutic approach to accessing the latent/ unconscious/hidden meanings of narrative through interpretation…Freud, the master of interpretation, did not arise in a vacuum. The Talmudic mode of thought became the ingrained model of the Jewish psyche, the intimacy and identity which Freud so keenly felt…For both Freud and the Rabbis, interpretation was the preeminent mode of knowing, applicable in every context and to every idea.
>
> (p. 207)

Sigmund Freud died in London on 23 September 1938. It was Yom Kippur, the holiest day of the Jewish calendar, and a year before the outbreak of the Second World War; when Nazi Germany was moving inexorably towards its 'final solution' of the 'Jewish question', the culmination of the anti-Jewish hatred which Freud knew so well.

The Development of Humanistic Psychotherapy

Following the Holocaust and the eventual defeat of fascism, Jewish men and women, such as Heinz Kohut, Otto Kernberg and Margaret Mahler, continued to be at the forefront of developments in psychoanalysis and psychotherapy. Other Jewish clinicians and writers, faithful to the humanism of Freud and the earlier generation of psychoanalysts noted by Dennis B. Klein (1985, pp. 148–150), moved on from classical psychoanalysis, responding to the tumultuous times, by promoting and integrating the values of humanism in new theories and paths for psychotherapy. In Chapters 3 and 4, I refer to the importance of Buber's Judaic-existential humanism in his conception of dialogue and meeting in the practice of psychotherapy. He also influenced the work of Erich Fromm.

Erich Fromm, a Jewish psychoanalyst who fled Nazi Germany for the USA, drew upon his Judaic background and study of the Torah, in the development of a secular humanistic philosophy and model. In this respect, the Judaic covenant between God and humankind was of great significance, involving the agency of humanity to challenge and argue with God. Fromm published several books which have been influential in the development of psychotherapy, such as 'Fear of Freedom', 'To Have or To Be' and 'The Art of Loving', and wrote:

> Is it surprising that the prophetic vison of a united peaceful mankind, found fertile soil among the Jews and was never forgotten. Is it surprising that when the walls of the ghettos fell, Jews in disproportionately numbers were among those who proclaimed the ideals of internationalism, peace and justice. What from a mundane standpoint was a tragedy of the Jews-the loss of their country and their state-from the humanist standpoint was their greatest blessing: being

among the suffering and despised, they were able to develop and hold a tradition of humanism.

(1966, pp. 18–19)

Exploring 'psychoanalysis as a Jewish wisdom tradition' Seth Aronson quotes from Anne Frank's diary. It is a poignant illustration of the Judaic humanism to which Fromm refers:

> It's really a wonder that I haven't dropped all my ideals, because they seem so absurd and impossible to carry out. Yet I keep to them, because in spite of everything I still believe that people are really good at heart. I simply can't build up my hopes on a foundation consisting of confusion, misery, and death. I see the world gradually being turned into wilderness, I hear the ever approaching thunder and yet, if I look up into the heavens, I think that it will come all right, that this cruelty too will end, and that peace and tranquillity will return again

(Aronson, 2010, p. 323, quoting from the Diary of
Anne Frank, 1952, p. 237)

Abraham Maslow, a second-generation Jewish-American psychologist whose parents fled the pogroms of early twentieth-century Europe, was one of the foremost pioneers of humanistic psychology, which is concerned with 'growth and self-actualization' of the human potential, which he called 'this third force': 'a reaction against the limitations (as philosophies of human nature) of behaviourism and classical, Freudian psychoanalysis' (2011, p. 242); and I believe, a response to the darkness the world was slowly emerging from, following the Second World War and the Holocaust.

Further evidence of the Jewish contribution to the establishment of humanistic psychotherapy is provided by the fact that three of its four major modalities were founded by Jewish people: Gestalt therapy by Fritz and Laura Perls, Transactional Analysis by Eric Berne and Psychosynthesis by Roberto Assagioli (Carl Rogers established the Person-Centred model).

In this post-Holocaust era, it was perhaps inevitable for Jews to have been and be at the forefront of the development of modern trauma therapy. Here is a list of some of the women and men of Jewish heritage who individually and collectively have made a crucial contribution to the treatment of trauma: Judith Herman, Francine Shapiro, Peter A. Levine, Stephen Porges,[1] Gabor Mate, Rachel Yehuda and Babette Rothschild.

Summary

I am in awe of the work and courage of Sigmund Freud, his colleagues and their successors in the following generations of analysts and psychotherapists; the lineage, depth and profundity of the Jewish journey have demanded my offering of this historical and transpersonal framing of their achievements. Such a collective contribution can be understood as a process of soul, an alchemic-like transformation of the experience of persecution and oppression; for the manifestation and bequeathing of profound psychological understanding in the pursuit of healing and human advancement. I consider awareness of the human soul's capacity for endurance, fortitude and brilliance to be essential; amidst the overwhelming evidence of the hate-filled, destructive and disastrous aspects of the human condition, which spans our world. It is important for us to know this, as individuals and groups on our respective journeys, and for the philosophy and practice of psychotherapy, these being the focus of the rest of this book.

Note

1 Here is a link to an online conversation concerning the connection between Porges's Jewish background and his work as a pioneer in the field of trauma therapy: Jacobson, R.Y.Y. with Porges Dr, S. (2023). 'Judaism & The Polyvagal Theory'. https://www.youtube.com/watch?v=i5W4Sx4wtMU (Accessed 25 August 2024).

References

Almaas, A.H. (2004) *Inner Journey Home: The Soul's Realization of the Unity of Reality.* Boston, MA & London: Shambhala.

Almaas, A.H. (2002) *Spacecruiser Inquiry: True Guidance for the Inner Journey.* Boston, MA & London: Shambhala.

Almaas, A.H. (1988) *The Pearl Beyond Price. Integration of Personality into Being: An Object Relations Approach.* Boston, MA & London: Shambhala.

Almaas, A.H. (1987) *Diamond Heart, Book 1: Elements of the Real in Man.* Boston, MA: Shambhala.

Aron, L. (2010) Introduction to the problem of desire: Psychoanalysis as a Jewish wisdom tradition. In *Answering a Question with a Question: Contemporary Psychoanalysis and Jewish Thought.* Aron, L. & Henik, L. (Editors). Brighton, MA: Academic Studies Press, p. 16.

Aronson, S. (2010) The problem of desire: Psychoanalysis as a Jewish wisdom tradition. In *Answering a Question with a Question: Contemporary Psychoanalysis and Jewish Thought.* Aron, L. & Henik, L. (Editors). Brighton, MA: Academic Studies Press, pp. 313–328.

Assagioli, R. (1991) *Transpersonal Development: The Dimension Beyond Psychosynthesis.* London: Crucible.

Brickman, C. (2010) Psychoanalysis and Judaism in context. In *Answering a Question with a Question: Contemporary Psychoanalysis and Jewish Thought.* Aron, L. & Henik, L. (Editors). Brighton, MA: Academic Studies Press, pp. 25–49.

Buber, M. (1958) *I and Thou,* Second Edition. Edinburgh: T&T Clark.

Cushman, P. (2010) A burning world, an absent god: Midrash, hermeneutics, and relational psychoanalysis. In *Answering a Question with a Question: Contemporary Psychoanalysis and Jewish Thought.* Aron, L. & Brighton, H.L. (Editors). Boston, MA: Academic Studies Press, pp. 369–400.

Diamond Approach (2004) *Ridhwan Foundation Information Statement.* https://online.diamondapproach.org/rf-is-aus/. Accessed on 4 September 2024.

Diller, J.V. (1991) *Freud's Jewish Identity: A Case Study in the Impact of Ethnicity.* London & Toronto: Associated University Presses.

Ferrer, J.N. (2017) *Participation and the Mystery: Transpersonal Essays in Psychology, Education, and Religion.* New York: SUNY.

Ferrer, J.N. (2002) *Revisioning Transpersonal Theory: A Participatory Vision of Human Spirituality.* New York: SUNY.

Freud, S. (2005) *The Unconscious.* London: Penguin Modern Classics.

Friedman, M. (1985) *The Healing Dialogue in Psychotherapy.* New York & London: Jason Aronson, Inc.

Fromm, E. (1966) *You Shall Be as Gods: A Radical Interpretation of the Old Testament and Its Tradition.* New York: Henry Holt & Co.

Friedman, H. & Hartelius, G. (Editors, 2015) *The Wiley Blackwell Handbook of Transpersonal Psychology.* West Sussex: Wiley Blackwell.

Frosh, S. (2005) *Hate and the "Jewish Science": Anti-semitism, Nazism and Psychoanalysis.* London: Palgrave Macmillan.

Grof, S. & Grof, C. (Editors, 1989) *Spiritual Emergency: When Personal Transformation Becomes a Crisis.* New York: Tarcher/Putnam.

Handelman, S.A. (1982) *The Slayers of Moses: The Emergence of Rabbinic Interpretation in Modern Literary Theory.* Albany: State University of New York Press.

Hartelius, G. & Ferrer, J.N. (2015). Transpersonal philosophy:The participatory turn. In *The Wiley Blackwell Handbook of Transpersonal Psychology.* Friedman, H. & Hartelius, G. (Editors). West Sussex:Wiley Blackwell.

Huxley, A. (1945) *The Perennial Philosophy.* New York: Harper Perennial Modern Classics.

Hycner, R. & Jacobs, L. (1995) *The Healing Relationship in Gestalt Therapy: A Dialogic/Self Psychology Approach.* New York: Gestalt Journal Press.

Hycner, R. (1993) *Between Person and Person: Toward a Dialogical Psychotherapy.* New York: Gestalt Journal Press.

Jennings, J. & Jennings, J. (1993) "I knew the method": The unseen Midrashic origins of Freud's psychoanalysis. In: *Journal of Psychology and Judaism* 1993, Vol. 17, pp. 51–74.

Klein, D.B. (1985) *Jewish Origins of the Psychoanalytic Movement.* Chicago, IL & London: University of Chicago Press.

Lancaster, B.L. (2008) Engaging with the mind of god: The participatory of Jewish mysticism. In *The Participatory Turn: Spirituality, Mysticism, Religious Studies.* Ferrer, J.N. & Sherman, J.H. (Editors). New York: SUNY, pp. 173–195.

Lings, M & Minnaur, C. (Editors, 2007) *The Underlying Religion: An Introduction to the Perennial Philosophy.* Bloomington, Indiana: World Wisdom, Inc.

Maslow, A.H. (2011) *Toward a Psychology of Being.* Blacksburg, VA: Wilder Publications, Inc.

Nirenberg, D. (2013) *Anti-Judaism: The History of a Way of Thinking.* London: Head of Zeus Ltd.

Rowan, J. (2005) *The Transpersonal: Spirituality in Psychotherapy and Counselling*, Second Edition. Hove: Routledge.

Schwartz, H. (Editor, 2020) *The Jewish Thought and Psychoanalysis Lectures.* Abingdon, Oxon: Phoenix Publishing House.

Starr, K. (2008) *Repair of the Soul: Metaphors of Transformation in Jewish Mysticism and Psychoanalysis.* New York & London: Routledge.

Washburn, M. (2020) 50 years of transpersonal psychology: Life of its current embers. *The Journal of Transpersonal Research* 2020, Vol. 12, No. 1, pp. 35–39.

Washburn, M. (2003) Transpersonal dialogue: A new direction. *The Journal of Transpersonal Psychology* 2003, Vol. 35, No. 1, pp. 1–19.

Washburn, M. (1995) *The Ego and the Dynamic Ground: A Transpersonal Theory of Human Development*, Second Edition. New York: SUNY.

Wilber, K. (2001) *Integral Spirituality: A Startling New Role for Religion in the Modern and Postmodern World.* Boulder, CO: Integral Books.

Wilber, K. (2000) *Integral Psychology: Consciousness, Spirit, Psychology, Therapy.* Boston, CO: Shambhala.

Chapter 3

My Philosophy of Therapy

The Therapeutic Relationship, the Self and Trauma

In the Introduction to this book, I provided an outline of my conception of psychotherapy and the treatment of trauma as a relationship for healing and self-realisation that holds and includes the relational, intrapsychic, transpersonal and transgenerational dimensions of human experience. In this chapter, I describe the philosophy of therapy with which I meet and work with clients.

The addressing of complex and transgenerational trauma and the uncovering and processing of difficult issues requires a person's engagement with the depths of their psyche. As I will discuss in Chapter 6, the significance of transgenerational trauma is commonly hidden from our consciousness, and so meeting its presence in and effects upon our lives can be challenging. Such work may have a dynamic impact on a client's experience of the self, which they will need to reflect upon and discuss with me. Thus, my capacity as a therapist for philosophical conversations with them concerning ontology and the process of psychotherapy is crucial within our shared and profound endeavour.

The Therapeutic Relationship

I hold an approach to the therapeutic relationship drawn from Martin Buber's religious dual concept of 'I-Thou' and 'I-It' relating (1958). An 'I-Thou attitude' (Hycner & Jacobs, 1995) is a commitment to engage with the immanence of the divine within the client and between us, being aware they 'are not a thing among things' (1958, p. 21) and that 'in each *Thou* we address the eternal *Thou*' (1958, p. 19). In this way, I orient for contact and a relationship between our two souls, for a journey of exploration and healing to be formed, informed and unfold. The 'I-It' (an instrumental objectifying mode of relating) is also an integral aspect of the therapeutic relationship, for consideration of a client's therapeutic needs with concepts and theory. Thus, in service to the client as Thou, I am required to consciously move between 'I-Thou' and 'I-It' relating, drawing upon concepts from psychotherapeutic theories to be used in dedication to the needs of the person. Of this dynamic, Buber writes: 'The particular *It*, by entering the relational event, may become a *Thou*' (1958, p. 50).

This way, through contact, engagement and reflection, an approach and plan will shape and evolve. My reflection and analysis may lead to either continuing

DOI: 10.4324/9781003456438-4

exploration with the client in a dialogue of increasing depth and intensity with respect to their issues or towards my employing a trauma-informed approach. The theoretical and practical aspects of the therapeutic process will be attended to and explored in Chapters 4, 5, 6, 7 and 9 and illustrated through case studies of my work with clients.

The Self and Personality

In Chapter 1, I described my personal journey through which my understanding of the self and psychological healing was formed. In psychotherapy, one's perspective needs to be available for reflection and discussion, and it is essential to be open concerning both the source and nature of the a priori and metaphysical beliefs underlying one's philosophy and approach. I agree with Robin S. Brown's epistemological assertion that all forms of knowledge hold them, explicitly or implicitly,[1] and that in this respect when metaphysics is repressed it will return 'as fundamentalism-whether religious or secular' (2017, p. 13) to impede dialogue and the phenomenological exploration at the heart of a therapeutic process.

I hold a metaphysical conception of the self as an individual and unique manifestation from 'The ground of true nature', which 'is one unified field that underlies and constitutes all existence' (Almaas, 2004, p. 263)… 'a true and timeless self, an Essential Self, a Self that is not constructed in early life…' (Almaas, 1988, p. 265). This is a conception of the self as an individual expression of and from the ground of being, into which all eventually dissolves.

In his dialogue with Carl Rogers (the founder of person-centred therapy), Buber emphasised the distinction between the individual and their potential for personhood: 'I not only accept the other as he is, but I confirm, in myself, and then in him, in relation to this potentiality that is meant by him' (Rogers Dialogues, 1990, p. 61). For Buber, the person is the realisation of the individual as someone '*in real contact*, in *real reciprocity* of the world' (1990, pp. 63–64)[2]. I believe such understanding is essential for the process of depth psychotherapy. Without it, we can be diverted from authentic engagement for healing and self-realisation, with a consequent exacerbation of narcissistic distortions in a client's relationship to self and others. I will say more about this further along in this chapter.

In the modality of psychosynthesis, I discern an understanding of the self which is comparable to that held by Almaas, with its concern for the 'Realization of One's True Self – The Discovery or Creation of a Unifying Center' (Assagioli, 1990, p. 24)…it being 'A method of psychological development and self-realization for those who refuse to remain the slaves of their own inner phantasms or of external influences…' (1990, p. 30). The latter part of the quote is similar to Almaas's distinction between essence and the personality, which is discussed below.

John C. Miller, in his exploration of Carl Jung's concept of the 'Transcendent Function' (the unfolding dialectical process of the psyche, which takes place between the conscious and unconscious mind) wrote that for Jung, 'the Self represents the center of all consciousness, both conscious and unconscious…the Self is also an archetype, the archetype of unity and totality' (2004, p. 70). And, in discussing the metaphysical depth of Jung's conception, Miller quotes him thus: 'Psychology has no proof that this process does not unfold itself at the instigation of God's will' (1955, p. 690)' (2004, p. 116).

With similarly poignant, transpersonal articulation of the human condition and its relationship to the divine, Buber writes: 'The development of the soul in the child is inextricably bound up with that of the longing for the *Thou*...Genuine understanding of this phenomenon can only be promoted if...its cosmic and metacosmic origin is kept in mind' (1958, p. 44). I hold such understanding as important with respect to the 'longing' of the client in psychotherapy, towards profound healing.

In contrast, a materialist conception of the self as a product of biology and conditioning restricts the scope, depth and prospects of personal exploration and psychotherapy. Robin S. Brown (2017) has observed:

> If we set out with an assumption that the individual is merely an expression of the material conditions from which he or she arises, then the patient's experience is inevitably demeaned as a mere epiphenomenon of genetics and/or social conditioning (p. 94)...

And:

> The notion of the reflective subject is seriously jeopardized in positing relationships as primary in the determination of the individual... Furthermore, the inevitable consequence of minimizing the role of the reflective self is that relational thinking finds itself falling back on biology wherever the claims of the social appear either inadequate or overbearing.
>
> (p. 55)

With respect for the mysterious and immanent qualities present and arising within each person, as a therapist, I need to be available to a client in their movements towards healing and the working through of veils of conditioning, trauma and intrapsychic defence. As children, we are dependent for our physical survival and psychological development upon the care, acceptance and validation of others. Our personality and social persona are both formations of beliefs and styles of relating patterned in infancy as creative adjustments to the demands, expectations and culture in which we find ourselves. Almaas's view is that:

> When a baby is born, it is pretty much all Essence or pure Being...Since most parents are identified with their personalities and not with their essence, they do not recognize or encourage the essence of the child. After a few years, Essence is forgotten, and instead of Essence, there is now personality...Although it was not seen, not recognized, and was even rejected and hurt in many ways, it is still there. In order to protect itself, it has gone underground, under cover. The cover is the personality.
>
> (Almaas, 1987, pp. 1–2)

Rowan, commenting from a similar perspective but with less compassion for this aspect of the human experience, wrote: 'The real self is a genuine centre, something like an internal gyroscope, independent of external influences. The mental ego is a false self, bound by roles and social influences and a prisoner of its time' (2000, p. 219).

Buber poetically expressed that: 'The *It* is the eternal chrysalis, the *Thou* the eternal butterfly' (1958, p. 32). This is similar to my view of the therapeutic relationship and also reflects my perspective concerning the personality structure and the self, with their intimate relationship and potential transformation. I understand Buber's 'I-Thou' (1958) as trusting in divine immanence and, as previously emphasised, the client's potential to be a 'person' rather than merely an 'individual'.

Concerning the self, it is important within the therapeutic relationship for me as a therapist to hold to the fact: 'The Thou meets me through grace – it is not found by seeking' (Buber, 1958, p. 24). However, through holding an 'I-Thou attitude' toward the client, I am in service to them for dialogue and exploration of their personality (formed for the protection of the self) – and self. This can encourage the client's soul to relax and open to the self, for it to arise and express itself through their imagination, 'peak experiences' (Maslow, 2011), heart's desires and creativity. Lily, whom we will meet in Chapters 5 and 7, healed from debilitating self-doubt and worry during our work together, to find a beautiful connection and flow from her creative imagination.

Abraham Maslow, while holding a secular, materialist philosophy, wrote of the 'peak' and religious experiences of self-actualising people as integral to their self-actualisation (Maslow, 1964). A welcoming attitude towards transpersonal and religious experiencing communicates trust in the client and encourages compassionate inner-encounter and exploration. I believe such steadfastness from a therapist for a client is important in their journey of recovery from trauma and the occlusion of the self to which Almaas refers in the above quotation. I also see it as an attitude, which on a socio-political level, affirms the struggle of people for emancipation, confirming their irreducible value as human beings.

Sometimes, I am required to guide and challenge a client when they interrupt contact and connection from the depth of their experience. Such interventions are made in service to their healing and self-realisation. These require my attunement to and balancing on a ridge of what is therapeutically tolerable for the client. However, in a well-formed therapeutic relationship, my falling off that ridge – either *via* confluence with the client's avoidance or by overwhelming them with too steep a challenge – may provide opportunities for reparative experiences in relation to historic mis-attunements. My welcoming and respect for their response to my mistakes can affect healing from the specific or cumulative insults to the self to which they have been subjected.

Such holding facilitates the exploration and processing of imprints, introjects and traumas to deepen inner connection and aid healing and disentanglement from historical and systemic family issues. As the self becomes freer or, using Almaas' metaphor, reappears from under its 'cover', this renaissance of personhood can be expressed in many ways, such as through illuminating insights, a freer range of emotions and heart-based desires. Such blossoming cannot be fully explained through reference to personal and transgenerational history, it is a manifestation from the mystery and immanence of being. In this process, I see myself as a supporter and companion in my clients' profound unfolding awareness and experience beyond the restrictions of introjects and the effects of trauma.

The Experiencing Self

In Chapter 2, I referred to Wilber's contribution to the inclusion of transpersonal awareness in the theory and practice of psychotherapy. The conceptual framework he provides in *Integral Psychology* (2000) aids understanding of the self and its unfolding process through its identification of different states and levels of consciousness, distinct foci and needs within pre-personal, personal and transpersonal levels of experience.

A valuable aspect of Wilber's model, which I emphasised in Chapter 2 (with Rowan's revised format: Rowan, 2005), is its identification of different states of consciousness and their differing orientation and needs from psychotherapy. This framework aids understanding of the ebb, flow and unfolding of a person's process and needs. Whilst our functioning is likely to be settled around a particular level of consciousness and focus for extended periods, we move between them. It is vital to be attentive to the figural needs of a client through therapy. For example, a cognitive behavioural type of intervention may be required where the intensity of trauma is overwhelming the person's ability to stay safe and healthy. In contrast, a client who is opening to an unfamiliar sense of self (including a 'Spiritual Emergency', which will be discussed later in this chapter) as they separate from their family's history of trauma may need encouragement and affirmation in becoming acquainted with this new experience.

Rowan outlined three 'Types of Thinking', which can help us discern and understand the level of consciousness from which a therapeutic dialogue and exploration is taking place: –

- 'First tier thinking' refers to the practice of formal logic as employed in the physical sciences, but of limited value for the understanding of human experience: 'It begins with the proposition "A is A" and carries on from there'.
- 'Second Tier' thinking is dialectical logic where 'A is not simply A'. This type of thinking is required for authentic contact and the practice of psychotherapy:

> It easily accommodates paradox and contradiction. It includes the doctrine of the interdependence of opposites, the interpenetration of opposites, and the ultimate identity of opposites... It is the land of I-Thou, not of the I-It... It is only at this level of thought that we can discover such ideas as the unconscious, subpersonalities, I-positions, "the analytic third" and so forth. This is

where we may discover the Shadow, and work through its ramifications: it is also the realm of openness, taken as a prime value.

- 'Third Tier thinking' relates to our experience as spiritual beings. Rowan observes it as:

the realm of the collective unconscious …also the realm of the subtle body, which is where the memories of previous lives are held… At this level we cannot ask the question – "Is it true?" We instead have to ask the question – "What effect did that have on you?"

(Personal Communication, 2013)

Alienation and the Self

There are consequences which can flow from an insufficient appreciation of and attention to the depth of our human experience. In my Introduction to this book, I referred to Bollas' discussion of the decline in introspection in Western society, towards a perspective in which psychotherapy is seen as a supplier of strategies and apps to ease discomfort without the need for engagement and deep reflection, where '…the psychoanalyst is morphed from a companion in exploration into a sage, appreciated in much the same way as one might be grateful for a good auto mechanic or computer expert' (2018, p. 64).

With such an orientation, we are likely to be prone to pursuing social conformity with normatively valued beliefs and objectives concerning who we are and 'should be', rather than self-exploration and healing from the trauma held in our bodies and souls. It is actually a state of personal and spiritual alienation for which we are seeking external supplies to compensate for its impoverishing effects. Such a separation from the depth of our being is commonly expressed through narcissism, which occludes the self and empathic contact with others and is marked by the domination of egotistic concerns with respect to our image and the external supply of acceptance and affirmation. Neville Symington understood narcissism as a turning away from depth and the 'lifegiver' within us, and thus from inner and relational connection: the lifegiver is 'a mental object that the mind can opt for or refuse at a very deep level' ('Narcissism: A New Theory', 2019a, p. 3).

In 'The Point of Existence: Transformations of Narcissism in Self-Realization' (1996), Almaas describes 'fundamental narcissism' as a ubiquitous developmental experience. He understands it to be the individual's drive to feel, see and have reflected to them their personal value and luminosity, whilst being disconnected from essence; bereft from the source, the ground of being:

Fundamental narcissism [is] the specific and most central manifestation of the disconnection from the essential core of the self, the Presence of being… Fundamental narcissism is an intrinsic property of the ego-self, which is the self as experienced in the dimension of conventional experience (p. 91)... The need for external mirroring feedback typically becomes focused on the need to be recognized as special and unique. This need reflects an exaggerated belief in one's specialness, which in turn reflects an underlying feeling of being insignificant.

(p. 162)

It is through reconnection with the depth that we begin to experience those qualities we have wished and sought to be present in our lives and become able to face and heal from trauma. Through contact within the therapeutic relationship, I encourage the client to connect with their depth and, in Symington's terms, turn to their 'lifegiver'.

With poignant appreciation of such issues, Symington describes the important, formidable endeavour in the 'job' of psychotherapy, to which therapists need to commit:

> ...to be possessed by the infinite, the ultimate, is sanity but to be possessed by a fragment of the whole, by a sensual piece of the whole, is madness...The job of the psychotherapist is to make contact with the infinite within himself. When he speaks from this then his patient also has the possibility of finding the root of sanity within himself.
>
> ('The Growth of Mind', 2019b, p. 94)

Such a commitment is crucial in work with transgenerational trauma when its depth and significance haven't been acknowledged and understood. In such circumstances, a client living with transgenerational trauma is likely to have a fractured understanding and experience of their self, with beliefs that they are fundamentally flawed because of their difficulties and oppressive normative expectations of themselves. Thus, we need to be the travelling companion Symington describes, for the depths to which he alludes.

Michael, who we will meet again in Chapter 7, lived with the transmission of Second World War traumas from his Polish parents, who were survivors of Nazi slave labour and a concentration camp. Entangled with the enduring terror, suffering and expectations of his mother, Michael had been unable to separate from her psychologically and found life frightening and forbidding, for which he felt shame and a personal deficiency. I sought to be empathically alongside Michael, sharing my beliefs and experiences with him in confirmation of his own. This was important in supporting him in processing the transgenerational root of his difficulties, which enabled them to ease along with the debilitating ruminations caused by his erroneous belief that they were expressive of inherent personal defects.

Personal Truth

In opening to an arising awareness from within us and through relationships with others, we can benefit from insights and understanding which aid healing and fulfilment. In this way, the occlusion of consciousness from preconceptions (sometimes manifesting as rigid ideologies) can fall away. Thus, we can awake for vivid experiencing towards the resolution of angst, psychological entanglements and trauma. Contact with new ideas and concepts mobilises us in feelings and thoughts towards enlivenment because dialogue, study and reflection are catalysts for experiencing personal truth from our 'creative core' ('The Growth of Mind', Symington, 2019b, p. 112).

One's dedicated attention to feelings, insights and imaginings can be a challenging process when we carry negative beliefs about ourselves from our personal and family histories. Consequently, we may have a propensity to suppress our capacity for self-reflection and the expansion of our consciousness and passively accept and absorb socially generated concepts, beliefs and values instead. It is an integral function of psychotherapy to support a client towards being free of unhelpful beliefs and injunctions emanating from their familial and cultural milieu, by holding and conveying trust in their process of introspection, reflection and self-discovery.

Within a therapeutic relationship, it is important for the client to be encouraged and supported in being grounded and centred in their experiencing and to hold 'negative capability'. This was a term used by the poet John Keats to describe the ability to dwell 'in uncertainties, mysteries, doubts, without any irritable reaching after fact and reason' (Keats quoted in Romanyshyn, 2002), which is important for the process of inquiry, digestion and change catalysed by psychotherapy. When we are open and reflective within and between the inner and relational domains, we allow a passage of self-realisation and the accessing of truth, which is significant to our lives. This is succinctly expressed by Jung in his essay 'The Transcendent Function': 'The shuttling to and fro of arguments and affects represents the transcending function of opposites…a movement out of the suspension between opposites, a living birth that leads to a new level of being, a new situation' (1957/1960, p. 90: cited in Miller, 2004, p. 3). I see this function of psychotherapy in Lily's journey. She emerged from the traumas of her family history and the first two decades of her life to open to her creative centre and become an author and inspirational teacher. The excitement, energy and freedom of her new way of being contrasted with the guilt-laden, self-doubting orientation she had carried from her youth.

The Challenge of the Emergent and Healing Self

In this book, I am articulating both the importance of appreciating ourselves as unique manifestations of being, and the need to be open to the transgenerational and transpersonal dimensions in the exploration of and healing from trauma.

Concepts (including diagnostic terms and categories) are important in psychotherapy, as I have described, with respect to the need to be open to both I-Thou and I-It relating. I consider concepts to have the potential to support or impede understanding and insights. The scope and practice of psychotherapy are disturbed and diminished when precedence is given to conceptual thinking over the fresh, alive qualities of awareness in our inner experiencing. This is because feelings such as desire, distress and anger are crucial signals which call for authentic, phenomeno-logical exploration and a practice of care towards legacies from past generations, childhood, trauma, neglect, rejection, abuse and oppression.

As therapy progresses (with deepening inner and relational freedom), issues concerning our identity, and personal and family history will move into the fore-ground. Carrie and I found that this occurred in response to her expanding assertion and expressions of self, personal presence and accomplishments. Through daytime terrors and nightmares, symptoms of complex trauma and internalised oppres-sion arose in juxtaposition to her progressive experience of self-realisation, self-actualisation and professional recognition. The theme of many of her dreams was of being at risk of murder by her abusive ex-partner and the rendering of danger for her new partner, closest friends and me. We found these to be confluent with the compound effects upon her soul of the abuse she suffered in her twenties and the fate of the Jewish branch of her family. The latter was an unacknowledged systemic trauma held within her family system.

Inner and relational (re-)connection brings intrapsychic challenges and tensions, as the person opens towards the breadth and depth of their being, and the living potential within and surrounding them. As a result, fear, anxiety and bewilderment can become pronounced as healing and new perspectives challenge and catalyse the vigilant, defensive beliefs and patterns of the personality. In *Trauma and the Soul*, the Jun-gian analyst Donald Kalsched writes about the 'self-care system' of the person living with trauma: 'The defensive system that "covers the abyss with trance" tries to keep the innocent remnant of the whole self from being further impacted by suffering-in-reality' (2013, p. 24). The intensity of the reaction to personal progress is likely to be in proportion to the severity of the challenges faced in childhood, concerning how much the person needed to retroflect – turn rejection, anger and hate inwards – sacrificing self in pursuit of safety and belonging (to family and social grouping).

Bert Hellinger describes the systemic pressures for conformity with respect to the drive to belong, which impede healing and self-realisation:

> It's gradually become clear to me that clients have a strong tendency to use their strengths to hold on to their problems and to avoid solutions. That has to do with the fact that psychological problems, unhappiness, or symptoms give us an inner assurance that we'll be allowed to continue to belong to our group. Suffering is the proof our child soul needs that we're not guilty with respect to our family. It secures and protects our right to belong to our family. Every unhappiness that's caused by systemic entanglement is accompanied by the deep contentment of knowing that we belong.
>
> (Hellinger, Weber & Beaumont, 1998, p. 223)

In becoming free from internal and social restrictions, it is important for people to encounter types of experience which might be outside of the range of those under-stood and accepted by this society's normative, consensus reality. These are paths of opportunity and challenge within the process of personal transformation.

Jung wrote in *The Red Book* of the riches and challenges in one's opening to experiences, outside of social norms and towards our finding a 'godly' balance:

> But know there is a divine madness which is nothing other than the overpowering of the spirit of this time through the spirit of the depths…The spirit of this time is ungodly, the spirit of the depths is ungodly, balance is godly.
>
> (2013, p. 150)

Richard House (2010), in his writing on this subject, provides the term 'Unusual Subjective Experience' (USE) – for appreciation, exploration and insight concerning hallucinations, the hearing of voices and other non-ordinary experiences that may surprise, intrigue or frighten us.

USEs arise when one's mind is challenged to open to a level or form of awareness to which it has been closed. On fleeting but significant occasions when working with a spiritual teacher, I found her image replaced by a vision of a Neanderthal being. I was especially intrigued because the identical figure had appeared 35 years previously, in my early experiences of personal therapy. Through inquiry, I found it was a channel and signal for my connecting more fully with an aspect of my personal power.

Carrie experienced USEs in the form of her brief sighting of non-material images and the frightening visions of melting faces. These occurred when she experienced an arising flow of previously suppressed trauma material for processing and following an accomplishment and or affirmation from an important source. They were significant, healthy manifestations, expressive of an intrapsychic dissonance and conflict between herself and her adaptive, defensive pattern of self-shaming and self-attack: her 'self-care system' (Kalsched, 2013).

We worked together on this frightening aspect of her journey, exploring the meaning and value of the USEs for her. Over time, the terror and shame the USEs evoked eased, and they became less frequent, eventually ceasing, as she moved into another phase of her therapeutic journey. Carrie's moving personal account can be read in the Appendix, 'Clients' Reflections'.

Stanislav and Christina Grof's positing of the concept of 'Spiritual Emergency' (1989) was an important contribution towards the appreciation of and respect for the needs and challenges we experience within the ongoing process of self-realisation. The concept refers to the emergent experiencing of 'non-ordinary states of consciousness' (Grof & Grof, 1989) towards spiritual unfolding and self-realisation. A client may need help coping with the arising of non-ordinary states of consciousness. Compassion and understanding need to be accorded to the normative and personal fears concerning the depth, mystery and intense challenge of this lonely journey, which are liable to be activated from them. It may be important for us to explore options for additional support, adjustments in daily living and helpful coping strategies with the client.

In this chapter, I have shared my philosophy of therapy, which respects and trusts the potential of the client and the therapeutic relationship for healing, disentanglement from the past and self-realisation. In the following chapters, I continue with an exposition of my approach and practice for the treatment of complex and transgenerational trauma.

Notes

1 Jurgen Habermas's 'Knowledge and Human Interests' (1972) is a work of epistemology which confronts this issue. He critiques 'Scientism...as science's belief in itself...the conviction that we can no longer understand science as one form of possible knowledge, but rather must identify knowledge with science' (p. 4); and argues: 'Objectivism, which makes a dogma of prescientific interpretation of knowledge as a copy of reality, limits access to reality to the dimension established by the scientific system of reference through the methodological objectification of reality. It prohibits discerning the a priori element of this system of reference and calling into question in anyway its monopoly of knowledge. As soon as this occurs, however, the objectivist barrier of the philosophy of science falls. As soon as we renounce misleading ontologizing we can understand a given scientific system of reference as the result of interaction between the knowing subject and reality' (pp. 89–90).

2 Hycner, in Hycner and Jacobs (1995, p. xxi) wrote: 'I have come to realize that what Buber meant by the dialogical is far more encompassing an approach than that which is emphasized in Person-Centred theory...It seems to me that a Person-Centred approach still fails to get beyond an individualistically oriented model of the self'.

References

Almaas, A.H. (2004) *Inner Journey Home: The Soul's Realization of the Unity of Reality.* Boston, MA & London: Shambhala.

Almaas, A.H. (1996) *The Point of Existence: Transformations of Narcissism in Self-Realization.* Berkeley, CA: Diamond Books.

Almaas, A.H. (1988) *The Pearl Beyond Price. Integration of Personality into Being: An Object Relations Approach.* Boston, MA: Shambhala.

Almaas, A.H. (1987) *Diamond Heart, Book 1: Elements of the Real in Man.* Boston, MA: Shambhala.

Assagioli, R. (1990) *Psychosynthesis: A Manual of Principles and Techniques.* Northamptonshire: Crucible.

Bollas, C. (2018) *Meaning and Melancholia: Life in the Age of Bewilderment.* Abingdon, Oxon: Routledge.

Brown, R.S. (2017) *Psychoanalysis Beyond the End of Metaphysics: Thinking towards the Post-Relational.* London & New York: Routledge.

Buber, M. (1958) *I and Thou*, Second Edition. Edinburgh: T&T Clark.

Grof, S. & Grof, C. (Editors, 1989) *Spiritual Emergency: When Personal Transformation Becomes a Crisis.* New York: Tarcher/Putnam.

Habermas, J. (1972) *Knowledge and Human Interests*, Second Edition. London: Heinemann.

Hellinger, B. with Weber, G. & Beaumont, H. (1998) *Love's Hidden Symmetry. What Makes Love Work in Relationships.* Phoenix, AZ: Zeig, Tucker & Co.

House, R. (2010) *In, against and Beyond Therapy: Critical Essays towards a 'Post-professional' Era.* Ross-on-Wye: PCCS Books.

Hycner, R. & Jacobs, L. (1995) *The Healing Relationship in Gestalt Therapy: A Dialogic/Self Psychology Approach.* New York: Gestalt Journal Press.

Jung, C.G. (2013) *The Red Book: A Reader's Edition (Philemon)* New York & London: Norton.

Jung, C.G. (1955). Letter to Pere Lachat, March 27, 1954. In *The Collected Works of C.G. Jung*. R.F.C. Hull (Trans.). Princeton: Princeton, Vol 18.

Kalsched, D. (2013) *Trauma and the Soul: A Psycho-spiritual Approach to Human Development and Its Interruption*. London & New York: Routledge.

Kirschenbaum, H. & Land Henderson, V. (Editors, 1990) The dialogue with Martin Buber. In *Carl Rogers Dialogues*. London: Constable, pp. 41–63.

Maslow, A.H. (2011) *Toward a Psychology of Being*. Blacksburg, VA: Wilder Publications, Inc.

Maslow, A.H. (1964) *Religions, Values, and Peak Experiences*. Cheshire: Stellar Classics.

Miller, J.C. (2004) *The Transcendent Function: Jung's Model of Psychological Growth through Dialogue with the Unconscious*. New York: SUNY.

Romanyshyn, R.D. (2002) *Ways of the Heart: Essays towards an Imaginal Psychology*. Pittsburgh, PA: Trivium Publications.

Rowan, J. (2013) *Three Types of Thinking*. Personal Communication.

Rowan, J. (2005) *The Transpersonal: Spirituality in Psychotherapy and Counselling*, Second Edition. Hove: Routledge.

Rowan, J. (2000) The self, the field and the either-or. *International Journal of Psychotherapy* 2000, Vol. 5, No. 3, pp. 219–226.

Symington, N. (2019a) *Narcissism: A New Theory*. Abingdon, Oxon & New York: Routledge.

Symington, N. (2019b) *The Growth of Mind*. Abingdon, Oxon & New York: Routledge.

Wilber, K. (2000) *Integral Psychology: Consciousness, Spirit, Psychology, Therapy*. Boston, MA: Shambhala.

Chapter 4

Theory and Practice – Relationship, Contact and the Healing of Trauma

In this chapter, concerned with my approach to working with trauma, I will first outline my appreciation and modification of gestalt therapy. With the changes I suggest, I consider it a valuable and fully integrative vehicle for trauma therapy. I then offer an exposition of my thinking about trauma and my approach to its treatment.

Section One: Gestalt Therapy and Trauma

I emphasised in the previous chapter two aspects of my philosophy of therapy in relation to work with trauma:

- The holding of Buber's concept of I-Thou and I-It as an orienting attitude to the therapeutic relationship.
- A Platonic conception of the self at the core of each of us, albeit suppressed and undercover, as a consequence of conditioning and trauma.

As a relationally focussed modality, gestalt therapy holds an integration of Buber's contribution. Lynne Jacobs writes of gestalt therapy as having '…purposely placed Martin Buber's philosophy as a cornerstone of its theory' (Hycner & Jacobs, 1995, p. 216). However, I believe the concept of self within gestalt therapy limits its potency and scope as a psychotherapy, and I outline an adjustment to incorporate the conception of the self which I described in Chapter 3.

Gestalt therapy is concerned with the exploration of our direct phenomenological experience, which includes the presence of the past within our beliefs and actions. Gary Yontef defines phenomenology as:

…a search for understanding on what is obvious or revealed by the situation rather than the interpretations of the observer…[which] works by entering into the situation experientially and allowing sensory Awareness to discover what is obvious/given.

(1993, p. 185)

DOI: 10.4324/9781003456438-5

A key concept in gestalt therapy is the 'cycle of experience' (Joyce & Sills, 2014) of the ongoing process of being in which need, interest and energy form a gestalt. A gestalt is a shape and formation for our here/now focus, with the potential to fulfil a need, desire or expression of self. Broadly, the cycle of experience is comprised of distinct phases:

- Sensation
- Awareness
- Mobilisation of energy
- Action
- Full contact
- Satisfaction
- Withdrawal
- The emergence of a fresh gestalt and cycle

In work with trauma, each phase will constitute an aspect of a person's exploration and processing of 'unfinished business' ('Gestalt Therapy: Excitement and Growth in the Human Personality', Perls, Hefferline & Goodman, 1951), this being the toxic legacy and effects of trauma in their life. In a discussion of 'The "Trauma" as Unfinished Situation', Perls et al. refer to its emergence, power and process from a gestalt perspective: 'Obviously the repressed trauma will return, for it is in a way the most vital part of the organism…it draws upon more organic power…the motion of the unfinished situation toward completion' (p. 297).

Integral to the framework of gestalt therapy is the identification with the client of their 'modifications to contact' (Joyce & Sills, 2014) from self, others and the environment within cycles of experience. These are:

- Desensitisation: For example, the loss or suppression of feeling in the course of a painful experience.
- Deflection: Avoiding or moving away from a gestalt, shifting one's focus.
- Projection: The disowning of inner experience, qualities, flaws and responsibility to instead see them as present in another or others.
- Introjection: Passively accepting, internalising and being directed by a belief imposed by other(s).
- Retroflection: The turning inwards of energy and aggression, for example, transmuting anger into self-blame.
- Egotism: A preoccupation and inner absorption that disconnects us from awareness of (and relationship with) others and the broader context.
- Confluence: Merging with another person (or persons) and losing connection with one's authenticity, vitality and inner-directed drive for being.

Each of these modifications is a way of managing trauma and its lasting effects on us and our relationships with others. For example, Lily felt guilt from the *introjecting* of the notion that she was responsible for her mother's feelings and *retroflected* anger and distress to instead experience them as guilt and anxiety.

We can understand a habitual pattern of a modification to contact as a 'fixed gestalt' (Joyce & Sills, 2014). In the context of trauma, a fixed gestalt originates from a 'creative adjustment' (Perls, Hefferline & Goodman, 1951) to provide amelioration of the overwhelming impact of such events. In enduring circumstances of risk and, or the lack of reparative experiences, these become incorporated within the individual's automatic way of being, for example, self-blame, dissociation, conformity, freezing, fighting or fleeing.

In work with trauma, by being alongside the client through their cycles of experience, one can enable a dynamic and compassionate understanding of the formation and modus operandi of these patterns for defence and survival. This, in turn, becomes a movement of engagement with their trauma towards a retrieval of self. That was the outcome in most of the case studies included in this book.

Integral to this process is the monitoring of my own experience to maintain presence and awareness with and for the client. Being careful and cognisant of one's capacity to move between different levels of thinking, sensing and understanding is essential. In the case study of my work with Angela, I reflect upon my interrupting contact with her as she sought to express and convey her suffering. With anxiety-based thinking and a drive to formulate interventions I hoped would be helpful, I regrettably distanced myself from the feelings evoked by our work together and, as a consequence, interrupted empathic contact with Angela's experience and needs during those sessions.

Gestalt Therapy as an Integrative Vehicle for Trauma Therapy

Gestalt therapy is an integrative approach to the human process, which can incorporate knowledge and wisdom from other models and aid personal integration. In the facilitation of the client's exploration and completion of fixed patterns of experiencing, orienting and relating formed through trauma, there are striking similarities between gestalt therapy and contemporary trauma models such as Somatic experiencing (SE) (Levine, 1997), Sensorimotor therapy (Ogden, Minton & Pain, 2006) and the Neuroaffective relational model (Heller & LaPierre, 2012). Later in this chapter, I summarise key elements of Franz Ruppert's tripartite model of the traumatised psyche (2007), which can be incorporated within the gestalt model of the human process concerning survival, adaptation and self-realisation.

Gestalt therapy, with an I-Thou attitude and attunement to the client's cycles of experiencing, is an approach through which the energy, pace and depth of personal work can be calibrated in accordance (and sympathy) with a client's needs, defences and general personal process. As I did with Lily, we can explore with the client their patterns of adaptation towards a relaxing of Kalsched's self-care system (cited in Chapter 3) and that which Ruppert terms the survivor part. As therapy progresses, the processing of trauma present and emerging from the individual's cycle of experience can take place. In this way, fixed gestalts and 'splits in the soul' (Ruppert, 2007) can receive attention for the easing of effects carried from the past.

Peter A. Levine has reflected that 'In a lifetime of working with traumatised individuals, I have been struck by the intrinsic and wedded relationship between trauma and spirituality' (2010, p. 310). I believe an adjustment in its ontology is required for the Gestalt approach to trauma to be unambiguously inclusive of the spiritual dimension to which Levine alludes.

An Adjustment: Gestalt Therapy and the Self

I value gestalt therapy as a vehicle for working with trauma and its effects. However, the therapeutic holding, which I believe is needed for the treatment of trauma, is restricted by its conception of the self. In gestalt therapy, the self is conceived as integral to, and evolving through relating and relationship, as part of the 'organism/ environment field' (Perls, Hefferline & Goodman, 1951):

This perspective is articulated by Perls et al in the following paragraph:

> Let us call the "self" the system of contacts at any moment... The self is the contact boundary at work; its activity is forming figures and grounds. As such the self is flexibly various, for it varies with the dominant organic and the pressing environmental stimuli... It is the artist of life... If a [a person] identifies with [their] forming self, does not inhibit [their] own creative excitement and reaching toward the coming solution; and conversely, if [they] alienate what is not organically their own and cannot be vitally interesting, but rather disrupts the figure/background, then [they are] psychologically healthy.
>
> (p. 235: The square brackets hold an updated use of pronouns I have inserted into the text)

This is a dynamic understanding of the self and its function and process in relating and relationship; however, it is a secular conception which does not appear to include the spiritual and transpersonal dimensions. It is a perspective emphasised by Peter Philippson, in his book 'The Emergent Self: An Existential-Gestalt Approach' (2009). He distinguishes between words which describe things and comparison words which:

> ...have no meaning at all except in relation to their polar opposites... The theory of emergent or relational self that I espouse says that "self" is the second type of word, a comparison with "other". With no other, there would be no self, and *vice versa*. It is always to this comparison that we are pointing when we speak of self. Thus self is not a "thing" or a given, but an emergence in a given situation.
>
> (pp. 2–3)

In Chapter 3, I discussed the problematic nature of such a theoretical view and outlined my conception of psychotherapy as attending to trauma with a metaphysical appreciation and understanding of the self. I believe this is necessary for the healing and re-connection to the self and soul, which have been affected by trauma and that cannot be understood through an exclusively autobiographical, relational or biological perspective.

The issue concerning the gestalt conception of the organism/environment field and the place and status of the self is highlighted by Rowan in his paper 'The self, the field and the either-or' (*International Journal of Psychotherapy*, Vol. 5, No. 3, 2000). He emphasises the importance of distinguishing the self from the ego, and, drawing upon Wilber's conception of the self, challenges the holding of a commitment to therapeutic contact and dialogue while discounting the centrality of the self in human experiencing: '...they think they somehow have to give up the idea of a central self in order to pursue the idea of dialogue. I am not quite sure why this is' (p. 221).

Robin S. Brown's words of caution, which I cited in Chapter 3, concerning exclusively relational conceptions of the self, are relevant here. I believe that in the absence of trust in the essential, irreducible reality of the self as a soulful, spiritual and ultimately transpersonal form, the profundity and depth of self-exploration and reflection will be undermined, thus limiting the potential of a phenomenological approach to support the re-emergence, healing and unfolding of the self.

Since training in Gestalt therapy in the 1990s, I have discerned contradictions within it, between a secular materialism and a phenomenological philosophy and methodology that leads to the spiritual and transpersonal, as evidenced by the work of some Gestalt therapists. For example, in stark contrast to Philippson, Claudio Naranjo, in his book 'Gestalt Therapy: The Attitude & Practice of an Atheoretical Experimentalism' (1993) asserts:

> ...the most distinctive features of gestalt therapy are, properly speaking, transpersonal...awareness is transpersonal...spiritual...
>
> (pp. 196–197)

Furthermore, he describes the self, in a manner similar to the conception I am offering in this book, as being distinct from the relationally and environmentally imprinted aspects of the individual's experience:

> The idea of being true to oneself implies, of course, the existence of a "self". If this term is to have any meaning, that must be the counterpart to character structure, the unconditioned-and, implicitly, the organismic.
>
> (p. 217)

Malcolm Parlett, the distinguished British gestalt therapist, highlights the tension within the modality to which I refer when he writes about field theory (an aspect of the philosophy and theory of gestalt therapy):

Writing and talking about the field can all sound too mystical for some....
especially so when people veer off into talking about using oneself as a 'resonating chamber'; being open to intuitive leaps and noticing extraordinary
coincidences... or even embracing a constellation perspective... Moving in
these directions seems to lead to a tipping point, when the needs for definition,
conceptual order, and consistent use of terminology cut in, and insist on being
paramount again... For many of us from time to time, there is an irresistible
temptation to delve into the arguments about what the word 'field' denotes: is
there an actual field of energy (as in auras, chi, the astral body)?...

(Foreword to Gaffney & O'Neil, 2013, p. xviii)

In those lines, Parlett has candidly articulated the issue for gestalt therapy – of
its phenomenological orientation, which leads us towards the transpersonal and
transgenerational dimensions, and to a countermanding secular reaction, which
assumes the exploration will render us in a place which is bereft of order. As I have
sought to demonstrate in Chapters 2 and 3, the integration of transpersonal understanding and a Platonic conception of self in psychotherapy are not 'tipping' points
into incoherence, but instead constitute a movement towards a holistic perspective
and approach.

We can see the potential (to repeat my quote from Parlett, with 'definition [and]
conceptual order') for gestalt therapy to hold the transpersonal dimension in 'The
Healing Relationship in Gestalt Therapy: A Dialogic – Self-Psychology Approach'
(Hycner & Jacobs, 1995), where Hycner writes:

There have been a number of questions raised about this being a "spiritual"
approach. Discussing a philosophy of dialogue, talking about the "between" and
mentioning "grace" places my thought explicitly in a spiritual context. By spiritual, I mean a recognition of a reality greater than that of the sum total of our
individual realities, and of the physical and visible world. It is inconceivable to
me to steep myself in a dialogical approach without recognizing a transpersonal
dimension. I feel more and more that in my best therapeutic moments, I am present to, and sometimes the instrument of, some spiritual reality.

(p. 93)

I understand that the modifications I am offering for gestalt therapy will not be
acceptable to those who conceive of the self in the way Philippson defines it.
However, I believe these changes enhance the model's qualities for working with
trauma and free it to be an approach that includes unequivocally the spiritual and
transpersonal dimensions. The theoretical change I am suggesting is to gestalt therapy's concept of the organism/environment field by including the self as a Platonic
form – an essential manifestation from the ground of being, located within the individual and available for phenomenological exploration. In this way, we can understand 'experiencing at the contact boundary as [an] expression of this timeless,
Essential Self' (Personal Communication, Orlandi-Fantini, 2016).

This clarification can aid our capacity to appreciate and hold the traumatised soul and the occluded self towards its healing and realisation. I believe the beneficial effects are reflected in the case studies I offer in this book. The change also maintains the commitment and contribution of the gestalt approach to an understanding of the person and their life, to be one of process and relationship, as Yontef writes, within 'a field [which is]… a totality of mutually influencing forces that together form a unified interactive whole' (1993, p. 297). But it is now a 'field' within which the intrapsychic and metaphysical are unreservedly included.

With this formulation, I use concepts from gestalt therapy in the following ways:

- Alongside interpersonal processes, I incorporate within the gestalt concepts of contact, contact boundary and cycle of experience an awareness of the intrapsychic, transpersonal and transgenerational dimensions (explored in Chapters 6 and 7). I believe this is essential for the reach and depth of work needed for trauma therapy and, more generally, in psychotherapy.
- Gestalt therapy is dedicated to facilitating and supporting the exploration of the individual's cycle of experience at the contact boundary of relationship with the environment and other people. I hold the contact boundary to include and denote the intrapsychic, transpersonal and spiritual space between who we identify as I/Me – and the who and that from which we experience, perceive and sense ourselves to be separate. This is important because, in the process of trauma therapy and its recovery of the self, the contact boundary between the I and Not I (aspects of self and the ground of being from which we have been disconnected and to which we can reconnect) will shift and change.
- I hold the cycle of experience with its arising, completing and fixed gestalts as a concept that supports exploration and understanding of all aspects of awareness and being, including those that transcend time and space. It aids recognition of and work with hidden transgenerational entanglements and traumas. This is explored further in Chapter 6 and illustrated within the case studies in this book.
- Similarly, I extend the Gestalt concept of modifications to contact, which identifies the ways we (consciously and unconsciously) manage, adapt to and adjust our experience of relationships and the environment; to include the dynamics of the self and arising aspects of conscious, imaginal and transpersonal experiencing.

With support from this framework, I share my thoughts about trauma and its treatment in the next section.

Section Two: Trauma and the Healing Process

It is important to recognise that traumas from overwhelming events and circumstances are unavoidable aspects of life. The forms of trauma which we take to therapy are causes of both deep suffering and alienation from the qualities of self, which enable a fulfilling life.

Trauma as consequences of neglect, abuse, violence and oppression in its myriad relational, social and political forms make life a terrible ordeal and are also symptomatic of our collective human condition. I consider my work with clients as a collaboration, with the presence and interaction between our respective histories and journeys of soul. I believe that to be openly met in this way by another person, in our suffering and its often-bewildering expressions and forms, is healing for the wounds and ruptures we carry, individually and collectively.

In an initial session with a client, I describe my soul-based philosophy and approach to help them make an informed decision with respect to commencing sessions with me. I believe trauma therapy is a process of soul for a movement towards wholeness, individually and collectively, with the inclusion and integration of the potential and qualities of the self. Thus, I strive to practise with that essential trust to hold, meet and reflect with the client in a manner that confirms their self and ultimate wholeness. I share with Levine the belief that where there is severe trauma: '…yet still, the smouldering flame of the deep self can miraculously reignite, given the right opportunity and carefully calibrated support' (2010, p. 192).

People who come to therapy for the treatment of trauma will have suffered overwhelming shocks to their functioning and orientation, causing the task of self-exploration and healing to take them along difficult paths they would not have otherwise travelled. So, to meet with a person living with trauma in their soul and body is an intimate and profound experience. In this regard, I value the cautionary insight offered by Davoine and Gaudilliere to all of us who work in this field: 'A natural – or, rather, social-inclination'…. 'distances everyone from the impressive knowledge of the Real these patients bring with them' (2004, p. 137). I concur, with the understanding that we will fail a client if our reaction to their sharing and transmission of suffering is one of detachment, and in this way, subject them to an experience of shaming and aloneness-pain (sadly a likely repeat of that endured both from and following a trauma). I believe such instances of one's withdrawal as a therapist from engagement with a client indicate the active presence of trauma within us, constituting an interruption of contact with them *via* egotism, projection and or deflection. Following such an occurrence, my self-reflection, clinical supervision and personal therapy are imperative for exploration, analysis, and a re-attunement with the client: As a therapist, I must meet with a client with humility, awareness and self-reflection.

I practise 'inclusion', with the understanding described by Yontef as 'feeling into the other's view while maintaining the sense of yourself…[seeing] the world for a moment as fully as possible through the other's eyes' (1993, p. 36). This allows the client's expression of their experience to enter me, with and through the different dimensions (including the transpersonal and transgenerational) of our explorations. I respect the primacy of the relationship field my client and I form together, with appreciation that a precipitative use of concepts (and their arbitrary parameters) can interrupt my attunement with them: It is crucial to be open to the emergence of helpful responses and interventions which arise from within our interactions. As I have stated above, where there are breaks and interruptions in my attunement, these call for self-reflection and, where necessary, exploration in supervision and personal therapy. It could be that trauma, as a configuring energy in the process of contact with the client, is having the effect of narrowing my consciousness, symptomatic of shock and dissociation. I again think of my work with Angela and my mis-attuned reaction to her intense suffering.

As part of my commitment to this work, I will draw upon contemporary approaches to trauma when they align with a client's needs as manifested in their gestalt cycle of experience. Thus, I have trained in Eye Movement Desensitisation and Reprocessing (EMDR), the Comprehensive Resource Model (CRM), Lifespan Integration, Deep Brain Reorienting (DBR) and studied and experienced Somatic Experiencing (SE) as a client for several years. I provide a description of some of the key features and use of EMDR and CRM in Chapter 9, concerning my work with Carrie. What I believe is of paramount importance is the guarding against introjecting (swallowing whole) modalities with a manual or protocol, giving them primacy and, in this way, disconnecting from personal engagement with a client. Thus, my practice of employing exercises and techniques is done with a commitment to ensuring that they are congruent with a client's needs and process. I include in the description of my work with Carrie, the realisation that giving priority to the use of EMDR and CRM contradicted her need to be met and meet herself through a dialogue of exploration, contact and healing.

Assessment and Safety

In the initial assessment process with a client, I seek to get to know, explore their ancestral and personal history and begin to develop an understanding of the burden they are carrying, which will help me to hold them and their family and cultural/ ethnic background in my consciousness.

I assess their capacity for engagement and safety within the therapeutic process through my experience of their presence and the information they share with me. This will include beliefs concerning their history and current circumstances, how they relate to me and to the environment of the therapy room, and details of help they may be receiving from other services, such as their doctor and the local mental health team. From here, I begin to form a sense of how we might proceed in our work together. Within my considerations at this point is the question of whether I feel confident as a lone practitioner for the therapy to proceed positively and safely.

Therapy involves a profound commitment from both the client and therapist, and it is crucial to respect both the potential client's need for safety and my own. To be misguided by personal grandiosity and or the individual's communication of personal emergency is likely to be a disservice and a terrible mistake. One needs to hold kindly to one's findings and, if required, consider which other available services would best serve a client and offer appropriate alternative suggestions. I offer these words in the spirit of humble sharing and support towards fellow lone practitioners facing such situations.

If a potential client and I decide to embark on work together, I will seek to facilitate our relationship through the approach I have described in Chapter 3 and above. The initial therapy sessions are significant in forming the therapeutic relationship and developing a sense of the type of approach that will benefit the client. It is important at this stage to help the client develop a sense of safety with me, the environment of the therapy room and the process. We will look together at how they manage risk and safety issues and explore challenges to maintaining personal presence and contact, such as from triggering of activations towards fleeing or freezing. I find the concept of the 'window of tolerance' (Ogden, Minton & Pain, 2006) between hyper- and hypoarousal can be useful for discussion and shared monitoring, with respect to a holding consciousness of the client's experience and providing protection from re-traumatisation (by becoming overwhelmed from an activated memory of trauma). This is with the understanding that if the client moves too far into either hyper or hypoarousal, the necessary therapeutic 'dual awareness' (Rothschild, 2000) of contact with me/the environment of the therapy room and the presence of the past will be lost. I often teach a client grounding and breathing exercises to sample and practise with me and use within and between sessions.

Compound and Cumulative Trauma

I have found that people often live with primary traumas from the transgenerational dimension and early childhood, which have combined with later traumas to compound and increase the complexity of their suffering. This is reflected in the case studies I have provided for this book, such as my work with Carrie. Naturally, the most recent traumas which provided the impetus to access therapy are likely to be the focus in the early stages of the therapeutic relationship. They can, in time, become portals to traumas and psychological entanglements which have been less apparent or hidden from consciousness.

Richard Erskine (1999) made an important observation concerning incidents and events which, in isolation, might have a minor and transient effect, such as a dismissive comment, mockery or inappropriate chastisement. However, if excessively repeated, they can form a sustained pattern of experience in a child's life, resulting in 'cumulative trauma' significantly affecting their sense of self and functioning in relationships and life. It is illustrated in my case study concerning Emily, in which a pattern of neglect and dismissal by her mother affected the formation of her personality structure and an occlusion of her sense of personal value and self.

Trauma which overwhelms the person's soul has enduring effects, some of which have been conceptualised as a splitting of the psyche and dissociation, to manage the psychological and spiritual devastation. Elizabeth Howell describes dissociation as 'the separation of mental and experiential contents that would normally be connected' (2005, p. 18). My approach is dedicated to meeting the person in their history, life and struggle and engaging with all that needs to be expressed and treated with compassion through our relationship. From the work of Pierre Janet, a pioneer of trauma therapy (Howell, 2005), there came the understanding that the healing of trauma requires completion of the unfinished process we carry from traumas (Howell, 2005), a perspective with which gestalt therapy is aligned, as indicated in my earlier quote from Perls et al. In Janet's terms, this constitutes the person's 'triumphing' over the impact, the profound shocks to body and soul they have suffered. It is a journey back from the 'retraction of the field of consciousness'

(Howell, 2005, p. 52), as expressed through dissociation, splits in the psyche and freezing of capacities towards wholeness and the accessing of their inherent potential for peace and fulfilment.

Trauma therapy has been identified by both Janet and Hermann (2015) as a tripartite process, with the phases named in sensorimotor therapy as stabilisation, processing and integration (Ogden, Minton & Pain, 2006). This framework needs to be understood in a non-linear way for appreciation and identification of the ongoing, shifting needs of the client as they move back and forth in unfolding journeys of exploration and healing. I hold it in my attendance to the gestalt cycle of experience within the therapeutic process.

The reader will probably be aware of the flourishing of neuroscientific research and literature concerning trauma, with some treatment models being closely identified with it. In my work and personal experience, I have been struck by the efficacy of approaches that draw upon neuroscience differently. For example, SE (Levine, 2010) and DBR (Corrigan and Sands: November 2019 Medical Hypotheses 136:109502): The former is aligned with the polyvagal theory of Stephen Porges and concerned with the process and healing management of the nervous system; and the latter with the process and healing release of pre-shock and shock trauma that has affected the person's functioning, *via* the superior colliculus and the periaqueductal grey in the upper brainstem in the midbrain. Despite their contrasting neurosciences concerning trauma and its treatment, both can aid recovery. They are effective through their different but compassionate ways of attending to the full depth and breadth of a person's experience and expression of horrors held in body and soul.

DBR

DBR is a trauma treatment invented and developed by the psychiatrist and neuroscientist Frank Corrigan, in which I have trained and continue to attend ongoing clinical supervision. I have found DBR to be a gentle way of processing deep trauma and complementary to my relational, gestalt approach, and I have integrated it into my work with some clients. I refer to DBR in some of the case studies in this book, and here, I offer a summary of how I use it in my practice, drawing upon: 'A randomized controlled trial of Deep Brain Reorienting: a neuroscientifically guided treatment for post-traumatic stress disorder' (2023) by Kearney, Corrigan, and colleagues.

1 Identifying the target: As my client and I explore a trauma, we will identify a recent or archaic memory, an 'Activating Stimulus' (AS), that represents the issue and process and activates an emotional and bodily response.
2 Orienting to the present: Using methods, we have previously found helpful for them, I lead the client to a grounding connection with the here and now, their core sense of self, and my supportive presence.
3 'O': Orienting to the traumatic trigger/event: I ask the client to bring AS back to the centre of their attention.

4 'T': Tension: I ask my client to notice any tension that emerges immediately in the head, face or neck. As with the whole process, my careful attention and attunement to the client are crucial as we proceed gently and slowly together. If they feel a strong emotion without first noticing a change and formation of tension, I guide them back to identifying any tension in the head, face and neck, as this is vital for the anchoring and safe holding of their experience throughout the process. Once the 'Orienting Tension' (OT) is identified, almost always in the muscles around the eyes, the forehead or the back of the neck, I prompt them to notice it, take their time and allow the opening of the next phase.

5 Shock and affect: With the OT located and anchored in their head, face or neck, I support the client to be with and tell me of their bodily, emotional and imaginal cycle of experiencing, which flows from their connection to the traumatic memory *via* the AS. I carefully monitor to ensure this process is tolerable and not overwhelming for them and that they maintain an anchoring sensing of the OT. I encourage the client to, as far as possible, resist the temptation to analyse that which is arising, as it can interrupt the process of release and the healing of the trauma that has been trapped in body and soul (I explain the importance of this in preparation for the use of DBR). To reiterate, my attunement to the client is vital for holding this delicate and powerful work to support and affirm the significance of their experience, ensure they are maintaining a dual awareness of the past and simultaneous present and not being re-traumatised or overwhelmed by feelings and memories.

6 Closure of the Session: In most cases, I have found the DBR process to come within the allotted time to a natural closure and the satisfaction phase of the gestalt cycle of experiencing, with a marked easing of the distress and pain the client has been carrying from the identified trauma. They often enjoy a sense of stillness and peace by the end of a session, with significant, new and profound insights about themselves and their lives, which sometimes have a spiritual resonance and depth. If the work is not complete, I will take care and time to support the client in reconnecting to and being grounded in the present moment, using techniques found to be helpful in our previous and preparatory work together.

If you would like in-depth information about DBR, I suggest: 'Deep Brain Reorienting: Understanding the Neuroscience of Trauma, Attachment Wounding, and DBR Psychotherapy' (2025) by Corrigan, F.M., Young, H., Christie-Sands, and published by Routledge.

Franz Ruppert: Splits in the Soul

For a broad theoretical understanding of the traumatised psyche, Franz Ruppert (2007) has provided a concept of it containing a triangular split:

• A traumatised part: Lost in shock, terror and shame, experiencing past traumas event(s) as timeless and perpetual.

- A survivor part: Vigilantly self-protective, with an avoidant orientation and defences formed to maintain separation from the trauma(s) and the overwhelming effects of those experiences. The power of this part is determined by the severity and complexity of the trauma(s) suffered and thus varies with respect to the extent it restricts the individual's capacity to relate and be.
- A healthy part: This is the part of the psyche that has remained able to relate to and experience contact with others despite trauma. Its range of functioning is limited, for which it seeks expansion *via* healing.

Each of the parts described by Ruppert is an aspect of a life with the effects of trauma and the need for contact (interpersonally and intrapsychically) in the healing exploration of our suffering, paths of survival and qualities of self. Such understanding of the psyche aids the therapeutic processing of cycles of experience (with concordant titrated attention to wounds and splits) and the enabling of recovery, 'triumph' and personal unfolding.

The Interactive Field between Therapist and Client

When trauma has impacted an individual early in their life, the healing process may require many years of therapy. This is because they will not have yet developed a capacity for 'mentalization' (Fonagy, Gergely, Jurist & Target, 2004) for relationally conscious and self-reflective understanding and management of their experience. In such circumstances, the psyche is likely to be split, with the effects of trauma managed through fixed gestalts (containing the modifications to contact of desensitisation, introjection and retroflection) by repression and dissociation.

People who endured a childhood overwhelmed by trauma and a lack of contrasting positive experiences are likely to assume their familiar sense of self and experience to be the natural and definitive state of being. In addition to Bollas' observations (to which I referred in the Introduction and Chapter 3), I believe many people seek symptomatic relief of their suffering without exploring their core experience as a human being: *Because they assume it to be immutable.* Sadly, complex, transgenerational and cumulative trauma requires therapeutic engagement and courage from both client and therapist, probably for several years.

Terror, rage, shame and confusion, being symptoms of trauma, are signals of suffering and difficulty which arise within us. At times, from the burning desire to be free of such feelings, clients are likely to feel frustration with themselves, the therapist and the process. It is also possible for me, as a therapist, to experience an inner reaction *vis a vis* the expectations I hold of myself, the impact of the client's suffering upon me, and my history. This can be understood in the terms of gestalt therapy as my becoming confluent with their projection, or psychodynamically as my experiencing a 'concordant countertransference' (Racker, 1982).

The Jungian concept of a 'collective unconscious' points us towards ways of understanding unconscious processes between therapist and client non-hierarchically within the gestalt cycle of experience. As an 'Interactive Field'

(Schwartz-Salant, 1995), it includes the transpersonal, the transgenerational and the occurrence of synchronistic events. Thus, I believe it is essential for me to have an inquiring attitude regarding relational and inner experiences, including those that are uncanny. The appreciation and processing of trauma can be aided by such reflection and careful inclusion within the dialogue, for example, in relation to somatic feelings of pressure, a narrowing of consciousness (Personal Communication, Dearden, 2023) and an interruption of connection with the depth.

I consider synchronicity to be an expression of the mystery and depth of our interactive and collective experiencing. It was something which Jung 'kept on coming across' when 'investigating the phenomena of the collective unconscious' (Jung, 1985, pp. 30–31). In Chapter 1, I recounted the extraordinary synchronistic event Robert and I experienced. During a Zoom session with another client, who had recently been bereaved of her husband of 50 years, a water cooler started to leak in her room, followed a few minutes later by the sounding of the house alarm. Neither had occurred before. In alignment with the intensity of my client's grief and pain and the depth of our dialogue, the environment seemed to be screaming and crying. I waited as she attended to the expression from these machines, and upon her return to the Zoom screen, we appreciated the moment, which had deepened our engagement with her pain of loss.

In Chapter 1, I also shared my experience of life-changing contact with the imaginal dimension, of which I have since carried a reverence for its potency and value. In Chapters 6 and 7, I explore and illustrate its uses for work with transgenerational entanglements and trauma. With echoes of Jung's model of 'Active Imagination' (1997), Robert Sardello has written of 'imaginal thinking' combining both cognisance within 'the mode of wholeness' (Sardello, 1999, p. 261) and the capacity for illuminating analysis and differentiation:

> Soul life does not conform to the ego's logic. When we attempt to understand the soul through ordinary logic rather than letting it instruct us in its own ways, we strengthen the forces of the ego and weaken those of soul life.
>
> (Sardello, 1999, p. 253)

This aligns with Rowan's identification of the ways of thinking (cited in Chapter 3), which support therapeutic and spiritual dialogue. The form and processes of deep trauma reside largely and significantly outside of conscious awareness. Therefore, expressions from the imaginal dimension, whether from dreams or experiences arising within sessions, are very significant within a collaborative addressing of trauma. This is illustrated in my work with Lily and Emily.

Exercises with the Imaginal

Reflecting its significance, the imaginal is common to many approaches in addition to the Jungian tradition. I earlier sketched its incorporation within my conception of gestalt therapy. It is also used for resourcing within modern neuroscience-based approaches to trauma, such as EMDR and the CRM.

Caveat: I have found that for some clients, this way of working is inappropriate because of their experiencing through their imagination of overwhelming activations of trauma material, which grounding exercises and the use of imaginal figures and resource structures will not ease. I reflect upon this in the case study of my work with Angela.

The specific form and intention of imaginal work concerning trauma arises from and develops through dialogue and exploration with the client. It will form and unfold from within the therapeutic relationship. Thus, what I describe below are examples which I believe are encouraging and helpful for specific clinical, intuitive and creative thinking for work with a client. They are not prescriptions for action.

- The Pleasant Place

    This is a visualisation, among others, which I learned through my training in EMDR (Shapiro, 2001). It can be soothing and supportive for a client at the end of, and between sessions, to experience through each of their senses a pleasant place or, if they are spiritually inclined, a place evocative of the spiritual dimension. For some clients, I have found a protective dome that covers the chosen scene, which may allow an increased feeling of privacy and safety. An additional resource is a stream of light falling from above, which I may facilitate a client to experience for a soothing touch to the parts of them that feel wounded and in pain. Again, it is important to mention caveats. Firstly, the client needs to choose a place free of negatively activating associations. Sometimes, people identify an attractive place, but that also holds connections with trauma. Secondly, it is important to watch for any adverse reaction and activation, such as the distortion or intrusion of trauma images and memories, which might indicate that the use of visualisations is not appropriate for the client, at least during this particular phase of their therapy.

- Imaginal Support and Exploration

    Some clients experience support, inspiration and re-connection with qualities of self by contact through visualisation and sensing with a being they admire from history, myth, popular culture or *via* their spiritual beliefs (e.g., a guardian angel). If this is attractive to a client, I will facilitate their seeing the figure (or figures, for example, if they choose a team of heroes) in their mind's eye, then sensing their presence (in front, alongside or behind them), and the commencing of communication, initially to check the figure is supportive and available to help. The client might like to pose a question to them from which they need guidance. We ascertain whether this is a helpful resource for the client from their direct experience of it and check whether they feel stronger or weaker during and after the encounter.

    Another exercise that can be helpful is the facilitation of the client to connect from an essential or adult sense of self to hold, communicate with and reassure a young, traumatised part of self. This needs to be facilitated slowly, taking care to talk and work with the experience of each part in the movement to and within contact.

Imaginal resourcing is central to the approach and procedures of the CRM in the treatment of trauma, including sophisticated visualisations of supportive inner environments for the healing process, and the reader can learn more from 'The Comprehensive Resource Model: Effective Therapeutic Techniques for the Healing of Complex Trauma' (2017) by Schwarz, Corrigan, Hull & Raju.

- 'Loving Eyes'

I have found this intervention, taught to me by Sian Morgan, a dear supervisor who died in 2022 and composed by Jim Knipe and included in 'EMDR and Ego State Therapy' (2008), to be helpful in trauma work with many people. When a young, traumatised part of a person's psyche is identified, I may suggest that the client looks at it from within their mind's eye with fondness and love. Frequently, this has a positive effect, relaxing the traumatised part's demeanour and easing fear, shame and anger. It can aid a movement towards connection and integration, with poignant imaginal work of dialogue and inner touch, with the traumatised part being held by the adult self, listened to and provided with sentences of confirmation and care. This can be repeated as a nurturing, healing procedure in successive sessions and perhaps used by the client between sessions as self-supportive homework.

An Illustrative Vignette

I used this exercise in imaginal work with John, a student of the Diamond Approach, who was living with the effects of growing up in a troubled, fractious family, within which the needs and qualities of his unfolding self were overlooked. John saw himself self-protectively holding the tail of a snake that was tormenting him. I asked if he could look at the snake with loving eyes. Being comfortable to do so, this began his movement into contact with the snake, in which the reptile communicated as a part of himself which had been made to feel he was 'nothing', and desperately wanting to be understood and free to go his own way. Relaxing into loving communication and acceptance, the snake became happy and friendly, and John began to experience peace and contentment. In the following session, resuming our work within the imaginal, he identified a hole in his chest, with the snake once more feeling rejected and exuding fearsome qualities. We repeated the loving eyes exercise, and John relaxed in a movement of healing integration. The snake, feeling free and restored through acceptance, fitted into the hole in John's chest. In the next session, he checked in with the snake and found the reptile relaxed and looking beautiful with vivid green scaling. John has continued his personal journey with an enhanced sense of equanimity with regard to the pleasures and challenges of his life.

If using the loving eyes exercise evokes an alienated, cold or otherwise negative attitude towards the part, this will be significant information about the client's inner process and history for exploration through conversation and within the imaginal.

- Supported Visualisation of Memories and Forthcoming Events.

A conversation concerning a significant scenario from the past or the near future can lead to the facilitation of imaginal support for the sense-experience of holding and personal agency and to see and feel a different and good outcome. Initially, I will ask my client about their emotions, feelings and the significance for them of the memory or scenario which has come to the foreground. We can then explore supportive figures and images that may enable them to feel secure and confident enough to proceed with this piece of work. If the client feels settled and comfortable, I then slowly facilitate their visualising movement into the scenario. Through each of the phases of this process, I frequently check with the client for each of their sense responses as they move through it. If the client moves out of their window of tolerance, we will pause or end the exercise with reorienting and grounding exercises. When they are ready, I will enquire about their reflections on the experience, its significance and any new insights which have arisen.

• Dreamwork

Working with dreams in the imaginal dimension can enable the expansion of personal awareness and aid therapy. Following a client's recounting of a dream which intrigues and mobilises their energy in sensations and emotions, I may suggest they envision and re-enter the dream from within their mind's eye in the here and now, for exploration and dialogue with and through its different beings and features. When we have reached a suitable place to pause or stop and re-emerge for full contact within the therapy room, I will invite the client to reflect upon the meaning this piece of dreamwork has brought for them. Examples of this approach to dreams are included in work with Lily.

Heart's Desires, Shame and Self-Protective Defences

In the following lines, Sardello articulates the heartful, soulful process, which I believe is integral to deep psychotherapeutic exploration:

> Heart awareness, heartfulness, locates being fully human within the soul and center of the spiritual body, the heart...In developing the capacity to creatively radiate from the center outward the holy, whole of the human body reveals itself as intimately united with imagination, creative presence...
>
> (Sardello, 2015, p. 1).

When the therapy has progressed to where a client's experience of self has deepened, I enquire about their heart's desires. A felt sense and awareness of these can help a client to connect with their personal essence, liberating energy and allowing a self-realising flow in their cycle of experience, which had been buried under the pain and despair of trauma. If a client is unable to sense their heart's desires, this can be an indication of an enduring alienation from the self. Where this is the case, exploring blocks, inhibitions and feelings of deficiency will be necessary concerning underlying issues, imprints and memories.

Where toxic shame arises (with feelings of self-disgust and worthlessness) about one's heart's desires, this may be a signal of a creative adjustment to cover up and protect the self. Bill, whom we meet in Chapter 7, found it very uncomfortable to connect with and express to me his wish for a relationship. This enhanced my appreciation and our exploration of the neglect, abuse and transgenerational issues that had been the factors in the inhibiting of his heart's desires.

With respect to survival patterns involving splitting and projection, obscuration of and disconnection from the self and accompanying beliefs of personal deficiency, I seek to facilitate, with a holding of basic trust and confirmation of the self, the processing of occluding and traumatic experiences for:

- A deepening relationship with the self, for realisation and fulfilment.
- Opening receptivity to insights, awareness and communication from within the soul, the imaginal and transpersonal realms.

I strive to hold a place of quiet attunement and inquiry with the client, appreciating the depth and challenge they are facing and, indeed, being quiet while present and open to what might be required of me. Or, I may be called to be active and talkative, mirroring, reflecting and affirming with a client who is experiencing the arising of personal history in their feelings and thoughts.

When a client reports powerful reactions to recent experiences, it is important to be curious about the themes and traumas that may have been activated from their history and experience of the wider field (including the transgenerational and transpersonal dimensions). In this way, contemporaneous reactivity can provide channels for deep and important work.

To follow and complement this chapter of theory, in the next, I will share with you three case studies of my work with clients who have lived with the effects of trauma.

References

Corrigan, F. & Sands-Christie, J. (2019) An innate brainstem self-other system involving orienting, affective responding, and polyvalent relational seeking: Some clinical implications for a "Deep Brain Reorienting" trauma. November 2019 Medical Hypotheses 136:109502.

Corrigan, F.M., Young, H. & Christie-Sands, J. (2025) *Deep Brain Reorienting: Understanding the Neuroscience of Trauma, Attachment Wounding, and DBR Psychotherapy.* New York & London: Routledge.

Davoine, F. & Gaudilliere, G.M. (2004) *History Beyond Trauma.* New York: Other Press.

Dearden, J. (2023) Personal Communication.

Erskine, R., Moursound, J.P. & Trautman, R. (1999) *Beyond Empathy: A Therapy of Contact-In-Relationship.* New York & London: Brunner Routledge.

Fonagy, P., Gergely, G., Jurist, E.L. & Target, M. (2004) *Affect Regulation, Mentalization, and the Development of the Self.* London & New York: Karnac.

Heller, L. & LaPierre, A. (2012) *Healing Developmental Trauma: How Early Trauma Affects Self-Regulation, Self-Image and the Capacity for Relationship.* Berkeley, CA: North Atlantic Books.

Hermann, J. (2015) *Trauma and Recovery: The Aftermath of Violence-from Domestic Abuse to Political Violence.* New York: Basic Books.

Howell, E.F. (2005) *The Dissociative Mind.* London & New York: Routledge.

Hycner, R. & Jacobs, L. (1995) *The Healing Relationship in Gestalt Therapy: A Dialogic/ Self Psychology Approach.* New York: Gestalt Journal Press.

Joyce, P. & Sills, C. (2014) *Skills in Gestalt Counselling & Psychotherapy*, Third Edition. London: Sage.

Jung, C.G. (1997) *Jung on Active Imagination.* Chodorow, J. (Editor). London: Routledge.

Jung, C.G. (1985) *Synchronicity: An Acausal Connecting Principle.* East Sussex & New York: Routledge.

Kearney, B.E., Corrigan, F.M., Frewend, P.A., Nevill, S., Harricharane, S., Andrews, K., Jetlyg, R., McKinnon, M.C. & Lanius, R.A. (2023) A randomized controlled trial of Deep Brain Reorienting: A neuroscientifically guided treatment for post-traumatic stress disorder. In: *European Journal of Psychotraumatology* 2023, Vol. 14, No. 2, p. 2240691.

Knipe, J. (2008) Loving eyes: Procedures to therapeutically reverse dissociative processes while preserving emotional safety. In *Healing the Heart of Trauma and Dissociation with EMDR and Ego State Therapy.* Forgash, C. & Copeley, M. (Editors). New York: Springer, pp. 181–217.

Levine, P.A. (2010) *In an Unspoken Voice: How the Body Releases Trauma and Restores Goodness.* Berkeley, CA: North Atlantic Books.

Levine, P.A. with Frederick, A. (1997) *Waking the Tiger: Healing Trauma.* Berkeley, CA: North Atlantic Books.

Naranjo, C. (1993) *Gestalt Therapy: The Attitude & Practice of an Atheoretical Experimentalism.* Nevada, CA: Gateways/IDHHB, Inc.

Ogden, P., Minton, K. & Pain, K. (2006) *Trauma and the Body: A Sensorimotor Approach to Psychotherapy.* New York: Norton.

Orlandi-Fantini, P. (2016) Personal Communication.

Parlett, M. (2013) Foreword to Gaffney, S. & O'Neil, B. *The Gestalt Field Perspective: Methodology and Practice.* Queensland: Ravenwood Press.

Perls, F., Hefferline, R.F. & Goodman, P. (1951) *Gestalt Therapy: Excitement and Growth in the Human Personality.* London: Souvenir Press.

Philippson, P. (2009) *The Emergent Self: An Existential-Gestalt Approach.* London: Karnac.

Racker, H. (1982) *Transference and Counter Transference.* London: Karnac.

Rothschild, B. (2000) *The Body Remembers: The Psychophysiology of Trauma and Trauma Treatment.* London & New York: Norton.

Rowan, J. (2000) The self, the field and the either-or. *International Journal of Psychotherapy* 2000, Vol. 5, No. 3, pp. 219–226.

Ruppert, F. (2007) *Splits in the Soul: Integrating Traumatic Experiences.* West Sussex: Green Balloon Publishing.

Sardello, R. (2015) *Heartfulness.* Houston, TX: Goldenstone Press.

Sardello, R. (1999) *Freeing the Soul from Fear.* New York: Riverhead Books.

Schwarz, L., Corrigan, F., Hull, A. & Raju, R. (2017) *Explorations in Mental Health 17: The Comprehensive Resource Model: Effective Therapeutic Techniques for the Healing of Complex Trauma.* Abingdon, Oxon: Routledge.

Schwartz-Salant, N. (1995) On the interactive field as the analytic object. In *The Interactive Field in Analysis, Volume One.* Stein, M. (Editor). Wilmette, IL: Chiron Publications, pp. 1–36.

Shapiro, F. (2001) *Eye Movement Desensitization and Reprocessing: Basic Principles, Protocols, and Procedures*, Second Edition. New York: Guildford.

Yontef, G.M. (1993) *Awareness, Dialogue & Process: Essays on Gestalt Therapy.* New York: Gestalt Journal Press.

Chapter 5

Lily, Emily and Angela

The first case study in this chapter concerns my work with Lily, who suffered toxic guilt and the trauma of childhood sexual abuse; the second with Emily and the processing of cumulative trauma from her childhood; and the third is an account of my work with Angela, who lives with severe complex trauma, in the past having been assessed as being close to meeting the diagnostic criteria of dissociative identity disorder (DID).

Lily

Background

Lily is an author, therapist and mother in her 40s. Prior to entering therapy, she lived with stultifying toxic shame and guilt rooted in family history, primary relationships and the experience of sexual abuse in her early teens.

Through Lily's formative years, her mother was insecure and emotionally fragile, which resonates with an opaque family narrative formed of anecdotes involving rifts and losses. As a consequence, her mother had a limited capacity for the consistent expression of parental love for Lily, subjecting her to neglect and punishment through capricious withholding of attention and care. Lily's father was a political refugee from an Eastern European country which fell under tyrannous rule following the end of World War 2. I write about our exploration and processing of Lily's transgenerational dynamics with her father's history in Chapter 7.

Her parents separated when she was three years old and with her young struggling mother resided for a time with her maternal grandparents. During this period, Lily's grandmother assumed the role of primary caregiver, providing support to her mother who slipped into the background.

Lily's mother eventually found a new partner and remarried. Lily adored and loved her stepfather, but in her early teens, he subjected Lily to a shattering trauma. He began to use a strategically placed mirror to look into her room and enter at night to sexually abuse her with touch, as she lay in bed. Following the second time of reporting this to her mother, a lock appeared on the bedroom door. This was done without an expression of care or acknowledgement of the abuse

DOI: 10.4324/9781003456438-6

from her stepfather. Her mother's failure to act against him, provide emotional support to Lily or speak/acknowledge the abuse left her lonely and bereft. She existed within the façade of a happy family until she was able to leave home.

At 18 years old, Lily departed for her university studies, carrying enduring feelings of shame, guilt and anger and a pain of aloneness for all that remained unacknowledged and unspoken. Following graduation, she began to develop a career in care services for children. Her experiences of childhood had seriously damaged her sense of personal value and experience of self, but along with her creative adjustment of accentuated attentiveness to another (her mother's emotional fragility), they constituted preparation for the practice of empathy and awareness required in human services.

Commencing Therapy

Lily commenced psychotherapy sessions following her enrolment on a course of training in counselling and psychotherapy. From our first meeting, I experienced her as committed and engaged, but also with an earnest desire to be liked. I felt warm towards Lily, but also sad, sensing her lack of trust in herself.

In the early sessions, Lily spoke of a sense of bewilderment concerning the intensity of her experience of angst and self-doubt. This disclosure, implicit of self-discounting beliefs, touched me as a beginning for our work with the suffering she carried in her soul. From here, it was important for me to affirm Lily's self and personhood. I also spoke with her about the significance of one's family history and encouraged reflection and conversation about this with regard to both her maternal and paternal lines.

We explored memories of her mother's unrealistic, guilt-inducing expectations and emotional abandonment of her, especially following her father's departure. As a child, Lily had made creative adjustments to adapt to her mother's behaviour, with a pattern of confluence (a merging in sympathy with her mother) and retroflection (self-blame, guilt and shame) as ways of avoiding blame and abandonment. Attending to this issue in sessions aided Lily's compassion for her ongoing fear of 'getting it wrong' and being subjected to another person's distress, judgement and rejection.

Trauma

Our exploration of memories and feelings in Lily's cycles of experience was a tender and delicate process of contact between us. It involved her courageous vulnerability in narrating key childhood events and her expression of distress, indignation, shame and feelings, with her nervously but clearly speaking out when she perceived me as being disinterested in her, just as she had frequently experienced her parents. For example, she voiced this on one occasion when I, affected by the energy of our interaction, briefly looked away from her and into the garden, and she challenged me; by which I felt catalysed with compassion and affirmation of her, which I shared. Through such work together, Lily began to progressively trust her personal experience and move out of confluence with her mother, and so deepen her appreciation of the disparity between the truth of her childhood and the sanitised narrative she had introjected from her mother (through which much had been obscured and repressed).

From her sense-experience, Lily frequently reported the feeling of a piece of wood present in her body from the neck downwards. I believe this was somatically related to the abuse from her stepfather and the shocking lack of action from her mother; these were combined in their deep and enduring effects upon her. They included toxic shame towards herself and her body and an agonising inner conflict regarding her relationship with her mother. As we explored together, integral to Lily's trauma pain was the memory (and persistence) of her mother's silence. I sensed a healing liberation as Lily felt and expressed anger about the wounds of abuse and abandonment with which she had lived.

Flowing from our engagement with this painful engagement with memory, I would facilitate her entering the imaginal dimension to see, hold and reassure the abandoned and frightened young Lily within. This work supported the experience of a wholesome balance between Lily's feelings and thoughts, and I encouraged her to practise it between sessions for a continuing and settling inner connection and support. We also used EMDR on a few occasions to aid the processing and easing of the pain of her memories and strengthen her cognition of having come through the abuse and subsequent years of torment, with belief and trust in her rights and self. Lily experienced a gradual easing of the pain of the trauma and the associated feelings of shame, and across the breadth of her life and relationships, she became more confident.

A Dream: Working with the Imaginal – A Renaissance of Creativity

Working with a dream, Lily found what she named as 'the missing piece'. The dream vividly portrayed her mother's insecurity and the presence of another luminous figure, which Lily identified as representing her own self. This brought the powerful realisation that early in childhood, with love and loyalty to her mother, she had held herself back from 'shining'. In the weeks following this liberating insight, Lily found within her imaginal experiencing a golden sphere, from which flowed soothing nourishment and supported her personal blossoming and creativity.

One day, Lily hesitantly shared two poems with me. This was her initial test concerning the safety in sharing her imagination and creativity with others. I felt moved and honoured. In time, a trust in and realisation of her talents blossomed, for her to become an author of books for children and parents, that support awareness, care and love. As we continued working with the negative imprints and introjects from her childhood, Lily's confidence grew incrementally through the many challenges involved in promoting her work. In addition to her work as a qualified therapist and author, she began to provide seminars in schools and to medical professionals, conveying the compassion and wisdom she has accessed through her therapeutic journey.

Motherhood and Continuing Healing

Lily, as a mother, is determined to provide an experience of childhood, which is a contrast from her own, for her children to feel safe and secure and grow up to be confident people. Within the therapy, we explored a tormenting notion: that she might be re-enacting her mother's behaviour towards them. This was activated by instances of feeling anger and frustration towards both her first two children, and especially her confident, challenging daughter. In our careful examination of these moments of intense inner experiencing, it became clear that she had maintained appropriate self-regulation and responsible parenting. I offered Lily the hypothesis that her experience of toxic guilt, formed as a child in her relationship with her mother, had transmuted and manifested as self-judgement and blame against her as a parent. Lily accessed meaning and relief from this interpretative intervention, and I facilitated her inner support through further imaginal holding of and dialogue with her frightened young self, again encouraging her to practise this between sessions.

Very sadly, in the following years, Lily suffered two late miscarriages, one being of twins, for which she needed an emergency medical intervention. With a resilience indicative of her psychological healing, a year after her second miscarriage, she gave birth to a healthy second son.

Working with a recurrence of her toxic guilt over the prospect of leaving her son for his first day at nursery, we used DBR (which I described in the previous chapter) for exploration and processing. In line with the procedure for DBR, I facilitated Lily's identification of an image of her leaving him at the nursery as the activating stimulus for the feeling of guilt and her sensing a place on her forehead for the orienting of this tension. She began to feel itchy, which was followed by the insight of having felt itchy on other occasions of feeling guilty. The sensation eased, to be followed by an unexpected rising in her mind's eye of the image of her maternal grandmother. Through feeling-sensing and a flow of memory and awareness, a few moments later, she received a timely, revelatory insight that the feelings of guilt she had been carrying originated from her grandmother. With release and relaxation passing through her body and a liberating inner sense of clarity, she exclaimed: 'The guilt is not mine!' It appeared that our years of dialogue, immersion within the imaginal and open attitude towards the transgenerational dimension had come together in fruition, to provide this liberating insight. The session, achieving a further easing of her toxic guilt, allowed a corresponding relaxing in her pattern of retroflecting energy and power formed in her childhood as a creative adjustment to her relationships with her parents and legacy of family histories. In the weeks that followed, she monitored her feeling and expressions of anger. Whilst she managed these safely, they concerned her, and she told me of a dream in which she kept a lion caged in her bedroom and felt confusion and guilt for having him in the home.

Commencing work with the dream, I offered the gestalt technique of two-chair work, for Lily to sit in a second chair to feel and speak as the lion. Strong feelings of rage and power emerged within her, and returning to her first chair, Lily expressed her feelings in a cathartic release of energy. She was moved by self-compassion, thinking of her suffering from her stepfather's abuse and her mother's silence.

a pattern of retroflection formed in the habitual turning inwards of bereft, lonely energy. This retroflection rendered her weary: A tiredness she remembered from childhood and now present in her life during our work together.

I was touched by the poignancy of her personal journey, her presence and the legacy of neglect weighing upon her soul. In our therapeutic dialogue, it was crucial for me to be present in my feelings and thoughts to provide Emily with an experience of contact, which contrasted with her childhood experience. This supported her undoing the retroflection of her life-energy and dissolving of self-suppressive introjects and involved my challenging and inquiring with her in moments when she voiced self-dismissal and self-judgements in attacks upon herself. They were manifestations of the weight of oppression carried in her soul.

In a year of sessions with me, Emily became able to re-engage with her creativity. An exciting idea for a new novel arose with both the research involved and its composition mobilising her energy. She became active again within the community of authors through conversation, retreats and workshops and decided to pause therapy with a view to returning at a later date.

The Second Phase of Therapy

Three years passed, during which time Emily's writing faltered again. When she contacted me to recommence therapy, the pressing reason was Colin's diagnosis of Parkinson's. Emily felt grief, foreboding and horror for the intense feelings of betrayal and rage she was experiencing towards her beloved husband for his affliction, albeit that his symptoms were mild. He had been advised that the progress of Parkinson's, or lack thereof, was unpredictable, his doctor's opinion being that he might well die of old age in his 80s. However, the diagnosis powerfully activated Emily's traumatic memory of her mother's excruciating expectations and dependence upon her, how unbearable they had been and the fear of reliving them with Colin. In her sessions, Emily's expression of these feelings allowed a movement in the gestalt cycle of experience to awareness of the mismatch of the past with the present, Colin being an undemanding, resourceful, empathic person, in contrast to her mother. This liberating awareness allowed Emily to look to their future with trust, in Colin and herself. She became free to think positively about her life, should Colin's Parkinson's progress and he die before her, forming a plan to travel around the UK in a campervan and write. She shared this with Colin and received his loving approval.

Fear, Family and Masks

In the foreground in this phase of her therapy was also Emily's relationship with her sister Mary, which caused her to feel a deep pain of loss, bewilderment and anger, and it became an important channel of personal exploration for her concerning her cumulative childhood trauma and suppression of self.

Emily reflected with me that Mary's attitude towards her had soured from the moment in her youth when she met and spent increasing amounts of time with

Colin. Over the following years, Emily had experienced Mary's behaviour as verbally aggressive, belittling and judgemental. A few years ago, Emily ended all contact with Mary because of her abusive and destructive behaviour towards both Emily and the wider family. This situation deeply troubled Emily, with a combination of bewilderment, grief and anger, viewing as a narcissistic bully, the big sister she had adored as a child.

Emily explored with me a traumatic event which began in Mary's Dubai apartment 20 years previously that had an enduring affect and resonance for her by evoking for her fear of masks and the shadows of her childhood. Present within it was the cruelty, contempt and jealousy Mary had subjected her to until Emily's breaking of contact: Mary became angry because of Emily's reluctance to be ostentatiously presented as her author-sister at an event she had arranged. She chided Emily for 'becoming too big for your boots' and condemned her for not following the fundamentalist form of Christianity she pursues herself. Without notice, Mary left Emily in the Dubai apartment, alone and devoid of her money and belongings. In shock, Emily had to find her way, in this unfamiliar foreign city, to a bank and the means of getting a flight home. Lost, bewildered and seeking directions, she found the sight of women in hijabs frightening and forbidding, which activated the terror of masks she had held since childhood. Eventually, Emily found a kind man who assisted her.

We used DBR to explore the trauma. For the procedure, Emily identified the activating stimulus of the memory as being lost and seeing women wearing hijabs and then located an orienting (and anchoring) tension at the back of her head. In the process of feeling-sensing-seeing, her focus moved away from the image of women wearing hijabs to Mary, her childhood and her lifelong fear of masks. This resonated with the frightening, intermittent inscrutability of her parents and elder siblings and their sudden switching of demeanours and behaviours.

Emily spoke of being deeply troubled by the perpetuation of abuse and suffering within her family of origin, and through the lines formed in marriage by Ronald and Mary, again bringing recall of the sense of darkness within her childhood home. Working with Playmobil figures to explore the constellation of her family of origin to understand her place within it, she saw her distance from other members whose drives and obsessions are alien to her (except the closeness to and care for Fred). The constellation painfully provided a visual clarification, distinguishing her way of being from that of her parents and elder siblings. It constitutes an imaginal resource and support for her deep self and onwards journey. I explore and discuss the family constellation approach to working with trauma in Chapter 6.

Permission, Self and Writing

Returning to investigate her inner restriction to writing and progress with the novel, we again explored her weariness and harsh self-judgements such as that of laziness.

I thought it important to contact the part of her who is resistant to writing. Using a repeating question with which Emily free-associated – 'What's good about Emily not succeeding in her writing?' – she uncovered self-denigration and a retroflection of her energy in adaptive accord with her lowly familial place as a 'skivvy'. The self-hatred which arose into Emily's consciousness was a shocking revelation for her, as part of a significant breakthrough in our investigation of this intrapsychic process, which deepened as she became aware of quietly holding the introjected belief, 'I don't have the right to be successful'.

In a subsequent session, after reviewing an early draft of this case study with me, Emily looked again at my hypothesis concerning the dream that brought her to therapy. This had a cathartic effect, as she connected with the budgie as a metaphor for herself, having previously understood it as simply about her creativity. Emily moved from shock to sadness and then anger, by which a mobilisation of energy replaced her weariness to feel 'bullish' in going forward with her life and bringing 'the little bird back to life'.

Arriving for the next session, Emily looked rich in life energy. Her eyes were bright, and she reported exciting breakthroughs in her writing concerning both the current novel and one she had left unfinished a few years back. Somehow, her self-exploration with me provided an opening for her to find the piece that had been missing for the book's completion, and she planned to contact her publisher to let them know the manuscript would be ready in a couple of months. Serendipitously, she also received unexpected affirmations concerning her talents from others, who urged her to put herself forward for public literary events.

Continuing this work in the following sessions, we explored her experience of shame with respect to her personal acceptance of her talents and accomplishments. Emily mentioned the feeling of embarrassment about 'showing off' by having on display in her home a photo of her with a pre-eminent, world-famous author. She curled and shrank into the chair as she visualised other people seeing this: She was 'frightened' and emphasised her sense of needing 'permission'. She remembered being fearful of making her mother unhappy, the anger of her father as he threw down the letter from her school informing him of her success in passing the '11plus' exam for entry to a grammar school, and when he received another letter advising him of the purchases he would need to make for her attendance.

With sadness and compassion, Emily expressed a wish to reach out to her younger selves. I facilitated her visualising, communicating with and holding her four-year-old self, who was receptive to and happy with this contact. This brought relief, and I suggested she practise this between sessions. She ended the session looking forward to working on her book the next day.

Through dialogue, dreams and work within the realm of the imagination, we are continuing to explore Emily's experience of self and attend to the oppression and injunctions that have denied her the right to enjoy life freely, create and be successful. Her work as an author is blossoming.

Angela

Her Background and Life

This is not a story of transformational healing, but one of fortitude and courage in living with complex trauma. It is also a lesson in humility and respect for the challenges that some of us face in the journey of our souls.

Angela was born in the early 1950s to parents who had brutal family histories of physical and emotional abuse and deprivation. She has attended therapy for most of her adult life, through which a significant degree of healing has taken place. Before me, her therapist was an eminent professor of psychotherapy whom she had seen for 13 years until he retired from clinical practice. This was alongside regular appointments with a psychiatrist, which have continued, as has her prescription for a lengthy list of medications. To date, Angela has been seeing me for 13 years. In our first meeting, she told me that her previous therapist had assessed her as close to meeting the criteria of DID, whilst having a degree of inner-witnessing and connecting awareness between different parts of herself, which held him back from confirming this diagnosis.

When we began our work together, the presence of ever-watchful, hateful and punishing gargoyles in her consciousness was a dominating source of oppression and terror. As she spoke, she would comment on their watching over and listening to all that she said and did, with the threat of punishment, such as making her blind. I understand the gargoyles represent extreme aspects of Angela's experience of her parents, their histories, beliefs and behaviours and her drive to comply with them. Within her psychological landscape, there was a 'dark' and 'white room' into which she would move when the terror or her feeling of 'wildness' became too strong. In the white room, there was silence, where she could not speak. We agreed on a plan for her to sign with me when this happened. One way she managed her inner torment was by cutting her arms with a Stanley knife, which provided release and relief.

While living with such suffering, Angela is a remarkable person who has helped hundreds of people, many at a low fee or none, through her dedication as a respected therapist and supervisor. This commitment to others commenced early in her life, with her mother and father.

Because of a mythological sense of its misfortune, her paternal line used the refrain 'The Smith Curse' for the marking of episodes of bad luck. Angela and her brother, two years senior, frequently refer to the curse concerning their experiences and fate. There are stories of ancestors having been war mercenaries, which are consistent with the violent dreams that torment Angela.

She describes her mother as being a 'clone' of her grandmother, a terrified person, bullied and shamed by Angela's grandfather and housebound by phobias and fear. In recalling her mother in early sessions, Angela spoke of her in both fearful and pitying terms about her panics, phobias and all-encompassing rituals: during Angela's childhood, confining, bizarre attention to Angela's personal care;

nocturnal housework, and a phobia concerning hairs. She was relieved when her mother passed away but also terrified of a magical retribution for feeling this way.

Angela has experienced gender dysphoria since before the age of five, loathing her female body and 'traditional' female behaviour. She became aware as an adult that one aspect of this condition was a desire not to live in the same gender as her mother, who was extremely 'feminine'. Several years ago, she was assessed at a gender dysphoria clinic and offered hormone treatment on the condition that, first, she lived for a year as a man. She reluctantly declined this offer because of concerns about its impact on her clients and supervisees.

The terror of death and many phobias has dominated Angela's life. Her birth, which had posed the risk of death to both mother and daughter, was traumatic. She describes herself as having lived with anhedonia since the age of 19. With her previous therapist and the early years of our work together, she described an extreme resistance to heating her house, even during the depths of winter. This was symptomatic of her identification with and loyalty to her father's stoicism and contempt of 'modern' comfort. Despite the overwhelming fear of death, in the early years of our work together, she experienced suicidal ideation, of killing herself by consuming a large cache of medication she had hoarded.

With a friendly, professional persona, she has veiled from people other than her therapists the reality of her tortured life, in which she has neither had an intimate adult relationship nor a friendship.

Angela experienced worry and compassion for the burdens of her father's life concerning her mother's issues and his struggles with money and work. Throughout her childhood, she dreaded his dying first and leaving her alone with her mother. However, she also vividly remembers fear and apprehension should he switch to being angry, with intensely 'red eyes'.

There were many rules in the home, including:

- Once in bed, Angela should never get out of bed, even to pick up a fallen pencil. She noted that her fear of punishment for doing so was worse than the horrific nightmares she suffered every night, from which she yearned for soothing. Shouting for help brought little comfort because she felt considerable guilt about interrupting her parents' nightly cleaning rituals (Her night terrors persist with violent, brutal contents, including murders and plagues of insects falling onto her and, in waking, a sense of the imminence of death).
- Angela was forbidden to speak to anyone about what happened in the home. This led her to form a habitual pattern of 'lying', which starkly contrasts with her painstaking honesty with me regarding her experiences, feelings and actions.
- No one was allowed to visit the home. She once invited a girl from school into the house. It is the only time she can recall breaking this rule, and she reflected that the act now feels inexplicable to her, given the gravity with which her parents communicated the rule: She remembers her parents' looks of anger and disgust. Still, she cannot remember what happened after the girl was made to

leave. Her sense of shame, dread, and inability to recall events following her breaking of a rule is a feature which is repeated within her narrative.

• Her mother's imposition of bizarre rituals regarding personal care, washing and managing of her phobia of hair. Over the years, her mother's domestic cleaning rituals became progressively more extreme. Angela would stay up all night helping, with her father catnapping on a chair before leaving for work the following day. The house was cluttered because of her mother's hoarding, and in some places, it was impassable, with the front door being inaccessible.

Angela recalls a crystallising moment at the age of three when looking at the night sky; she experienced the commencing of an omnipresent terror of death, which has dominated her life. A year later, her brother led her to escape from home. They were found and brought back. Again, she can't remember what happened in the aftermath. Early in childhood, she developed intense patterns of avoidance and ritual (such as checking public fire hydrant signs), by which I understand she sought to manage her experience of anxiety and agoraphobia.

Bound in fear and loyalty to her parents' demand for secrecy, in her school years, Angela hoped desperately that a teacher would discover her plight and enable her to escape home or remedy the situation by removing her mother. This didn't occur, and school was an experience that compounded her traumas at home. She was subjected to humiliation from both teachers and students, partly because of her attire, which reflected the family's poverty. Illustrative of the complex nature of her relationship with her mother, Angela would rush home from school each day to meet her, waiting and weeping on the stairs. Angela would then sit and listen devotedly to her mother. This was a precursor to her compassionate commitment to her clients and supervisees.

By her teens, Angela was a day-patient at the local psychiatric hospital, of which she has grim memories, such as being placed in the geriatric lounge where her paternal grandfather also sat.

In testimony to both her talents and grit, in her early twenties, Angela gained entrance to university, but the intensity of the trauma she was carrying caused this to be a disastrous ordeal which she had to end after a year. Returning home, her agoraphobia worsened, and she developed severe anorexia, necessitating hospitalisation when her weight dropped to below four stone. Angela was discharged when she reached five-and-a-half stone. For many years, she hid weights in her pockets whenever she was to be weighed. In the early phase of our work together, Angela expressed pride to me concerning her willpower, which enabled her to become so severely emaciated. She believed it to be an achievement in alignment with her father's stoicism and commenced a fresh phase of self-starvation. With Angela's consent, I liaised with her psychiatrist, and in time, the process and our concerns eased. She continues to exclude cooked and solid food from her diet and has a diagnosis of ARFID (avoidant/restrictive food intake disorder).

In her early 30s, in desperation because of her agoraphobia and anxiety, Angela approached a private Chartered Psychologist. This action generated acute guilt and shame as it diverged from the secretive ways and rules of the family, with her lying to her parents that she would only address the anorexia in these sessions. Her father drove her to the sessions, waiting for her in a cold car; her mother at home exclaiming that she had been 'abandoned'.

Angela believed that the therapist cared, and being 'naïve', she assumed that his stroking of her body under her clothes was a therapeutic technique, even though it left her feeling dirty and ashamed. After several months, with the dawning realisation that she was being sexually abused, Angela terminated the sessions. She never told anyone, believing this experience was a punishment for breaking the family rule of 'Never talk, never trust'.

A few years later, she felt able to try again and accessed genuine therapy – an unbroken process she has continued since. Remarkably, she studied for a university course in psychology whilst existing within her family's madness, was awarded a First-Class Honours degree and commenced her training as a therapist. Angela left home in her 40s, developed a successful therapy practice and highly respected place within the profession, and was involved in the establishment and management of a concessional counselling service for people living on low incomes. In time, she became a sought-after trainer concerning therapy for survivors of child sexual abuse. However, her unremitting existential terror continued, as did the absence of any relationship, friendship or social acquaintance in her life.

In her professional life, she conveys a warm and cheerful therapist persona, separate from the reality of her inner experience. This dissociative process, whilst it must affect the interactive field with her clients, does not appear to interfere with her capacity to be truly therapeutic. She has a strong reputation as a practitioner, and her services are highly valued and sought after. As described below, we have nurtured and utilised her therapist persona as a resource to support her and the therapeutic process.

Working Together

From our first encounter, I was struck by the intensity of Angela's suffering and her fortitude as she meticulously shared her history and information concerning her previous experiences of therapy. We developed a relationship within which she openly and frequently viscerally, expressed a volatile range of feelings and expressions, including terror, self-hatred and grief, from different parts of her fragmented psyche. In the early years of our work together, she found the gaps between meeting me extremely difficult, counting off the days between sessions and calling them her 'fix'. Through her gestalt cycles of experience in sessions, Angela expressed and explored with great intensity, with me striving to provide both supportive witnessing and therapeutic holding for her. Through experimentation, we discovered that her holding EMDR hand pulsers for tactile bilateral stimulation (Shapiro, 2001) at a slow pace was a little soothing and mildly beneficial.

Work with Parts of Angela's Psyche

In addition to the gestalt dialogue, we also worked with her fragmented psyche using various modalities. These included ego-state therapy (Watkins & Watkins, 1997) combined with a modified form of EMDR (Forgash & Copeley, 2008), CRM and internal family systems therapy (Schwartz and Sweezy, 2020) in pursuit of an easing of the tortuous conflict in her psyche that is symptomatic of severe, complex trauma and dissociation (Hart, Nijenhuis & Steele, 2006). This collaboration with Angela required my utmost attentive care, for which I took regular, specialist clinical supervision. Despite its challenges, her commitment and courage were palpable throughout: in the preparatory conversations, setting up engagement with parts of her psyche, visualising, my dialoguing with them and her and subsequent reflective discussions.

Angela composed and gave me Figures 5.1–5.3 (The latter comprising a list of parts of her psyche) concerning her inner world:

In Figure 5.1, her small, terrified child is hiding at the back of a cave, oppressed by the frightening figures of the gargoyles and the critic. This image depicts the crushing effects of the traumas she carries from her history, with her self-attacking adaptation and submission to the terrifying family environment (represented by the gargoyles and the critic). Angela impacted me by vocalising her child and vividly describing the terrain and experience in this horrific, imaginal realm: paralysed by fear.

- Helping her find comforting figures, represented by Clint Eastwood and Steve McQueen, took many sessions and brought a minor supply of support to the scared child. When I proposed that they move closer, the child's fear of punishment from the gargoyles became overwhelming, so she could only manage a visualisation of Clint and Steve standing by the entrance to the cave.
- The therapist is a male resource figure, drawing upon her professional experience and persona. We nurtured and continued to call upon him following the discontinuing of structured work with Angela's parts. He can provide support with a balanced perspective and holding for Angela; however, his availability is affected by the level of fear active in her at any time. When this is heightened, he becomes submerged and difficult to connect with.
- In Figures 5.1 and 5.2, her self-attacking parts (the gargoyles and critic) are depicted hating, threatening and deriding the child and supportive parts while proclaiming their disconnection from her as all-powerful, all-knowing figures transcendent of space and time. These are figures which, again, actually represent deep suffering, transmuted into fierce defence mechanisms of dissociation and inner attack – the 'self-care system' as named by Kalsched (2013), who I cited in Chapters 3 and 4. Through work, including my exploratory dialogues with them concerning their hatred of Angela and their origins, there was some minor easing of their power over her. She became a little freer to see past their preposterous claims of omniscience, to allow more consciousness of their function as self-suppressive protectors formed in infancy.

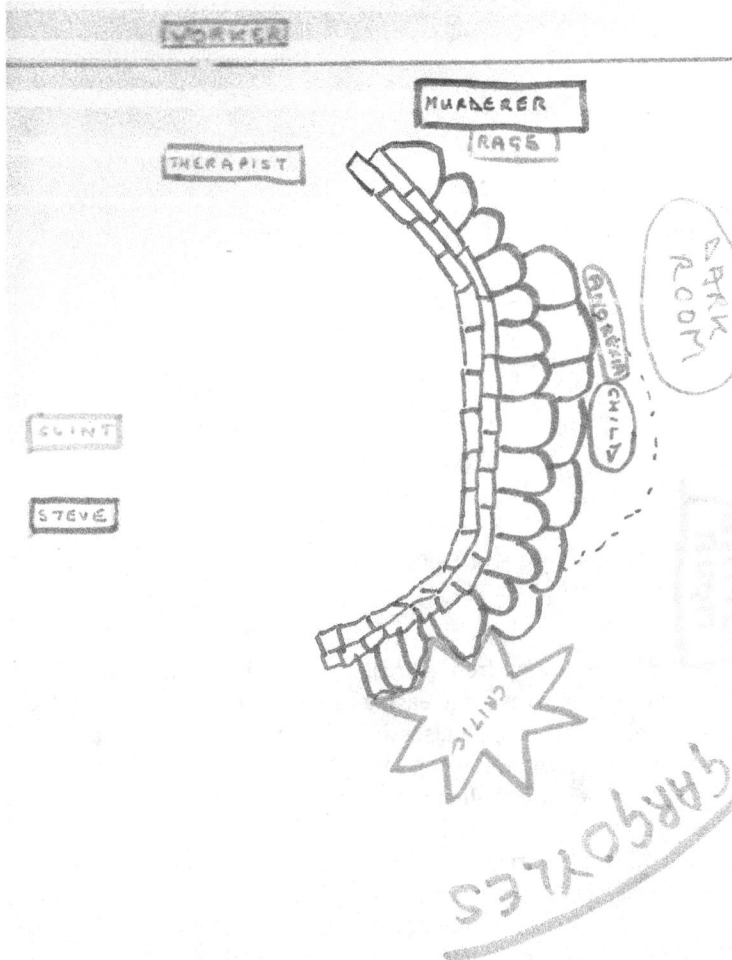

Figure 5.1 Angela's representation of different parts of her psyche in the imaginal context of a cave.

- Note the proximity of her anorexic part to the frightened child, which existed in confluence with the privations of her parents with a desperate holding of a residual sense of personal control and agency through self-starvation.
- Her murderer is the counterpart to her terrified self, being full of energy, rage and hatred towards the world – expressive of her suffering and holding the polar position from the other end, where the therapist is situated. The worker is placed in the middle of this continuum.

Concentrated work with Angela's parts took place in two phases of our work together, the first in the early years of her therapy and the second following

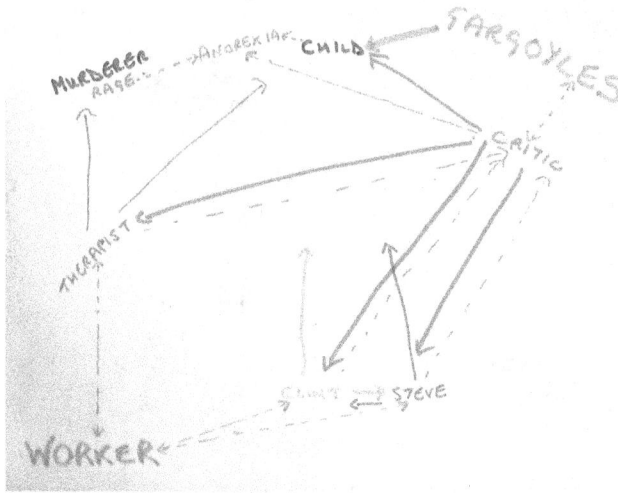

Figure 5.2 Angela's depiction of her psyche, lines indicating flow and connection between self-parts.

discussion after her returning from a break of several months for a back operation. As a result of both, there was some easing of her volatility and an enhancement of the presence of her core self within sessions, her being able to remain in conversation with me for longer without being overwhelmed by attacks from the gargoyles and the critic. However, the challenge and fear activated by working with her parts did eventually lead Angela, both times, to seek a return to a therapeutic dialogue, in which she could concentrate her expression to me of the ongoing suffering from her perpetual existential terrors. A priority for her is my hearing and witnessing her lonely torment, which is filled with the ever-present fear of death (e.g., from cancer or heart attack), night terrors and existential crises related to domestic and work issues, always with a sense of impending catastrophe. She endures these alongside the medical issues, she has been fated to suffer. These include three back operations (the hospital stays being, for her, tortuous re-enactments of childhood physical confinement, neglect and shaming), constant physical pain and the prognosis of eventual 95% blindness from juvenile macular degeneration.

Without a Safe Place

Perhaps the most significant challenge in our work together has been Angela's difficulty finding and experiencing holding and soothing, whether through personal contact or the imaginal and spiritual dimensions. The techniques for facilitating holding and support, which I have described earlier in this chapter, beneficial in one form or another for all the other clients I have written about in this book, were ineffective and triggered horror within her. For example, her love of dogs (the two

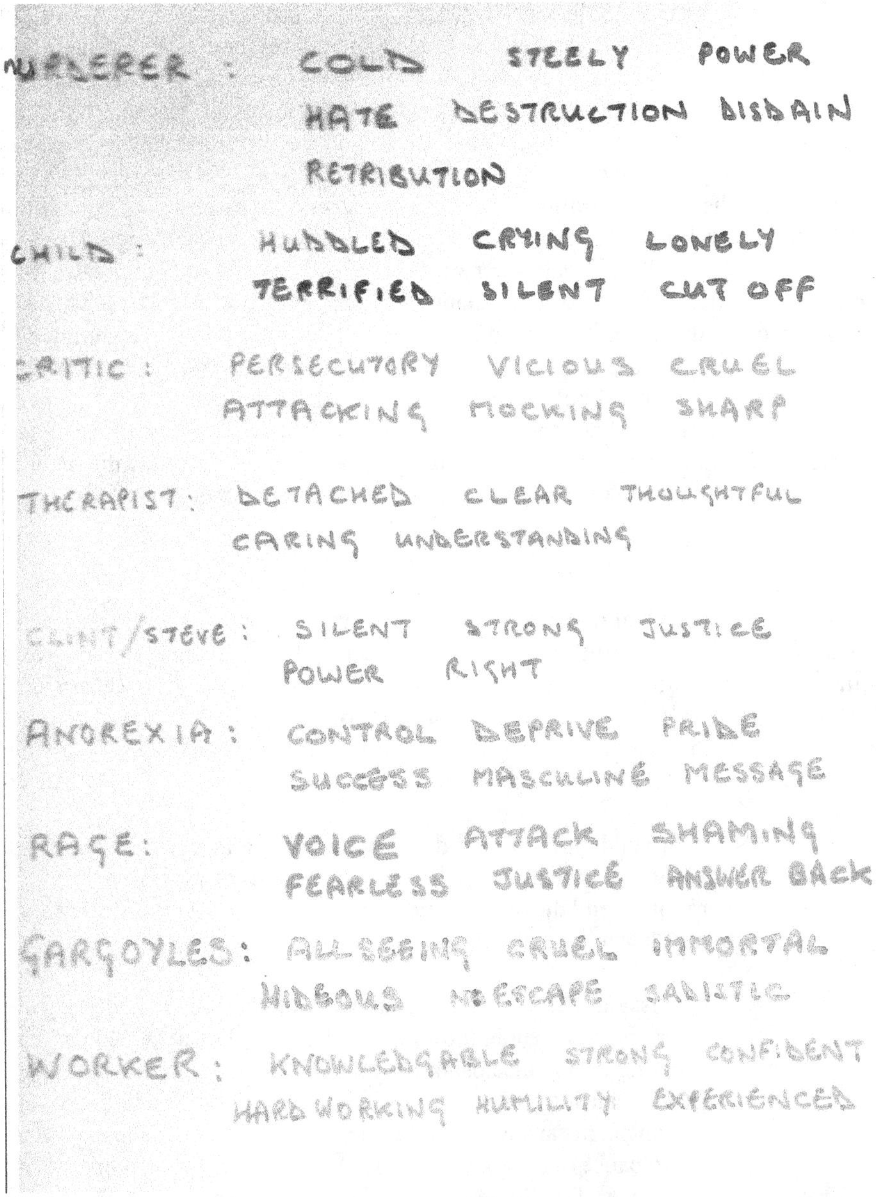

MURDERER : COLD   STEELY   POWER
HATE   DESTRUCTION   DISDAIN
RETRIBUTION

CHILD : HUDDLED   CRYING   LONELY
TERRIFIED   SILENT   CUT OFF

CRITIC : PERSECUTORY   VICIOUS   CRUEL
ATTACKING   MOCKING   SHARP

THERAPIST : DETACHED   CLEAR   THOUGHTFUL
CARING   UNDERSTANDING

CLINT/STEVE : SILENT   STRONG   JUSTICE
POWER   RIGHT

ANOREXIA : CONTROL   DEPRIVE   PRIDE
SUCCESS   MASCULINE   MESSAGE

RAGE : VOICE   ATTACK   SHAMING
FEARLESS   JUSTICE   ANSWER BACK

GARGOYLES : ALL SEEING   CRUEL   IMMORTAL
HIDEOUS   NO ESCAPE   SADISTIC

WORKER : KNOWLEDGABLE   STRONG   CONFIDENT
HARD WORKING   HUMILITY   EXPERIENCED

Figure 5.3 Angela's list and description of self-parts.

pet dogs she had earlier in her life had provided her with her most significant experiences of positive contact) encouraged us to experiment with her feeling soothing by looking at photos of dogs with me. Angela chose one picture that was especially pleasing to her. However, within the coming days, the image transmuted within her mind's eye to torment her, becoming a scene of the torture and mutilation of the dog. Symptomatic of her desperate lack of inner holding and safety, Angela has a collection of cuddly toys, which are not objects of comfort for her but instead purchased because she experienced a pleading from them for rescue from shop windows. They represent her troubled soul and that of her parents, in desperate need of sanctuary and love.

To address the transgenerational dimension of Angela's experience, in addition to Playmobil work figure regarding her family history, I also facilitated Angela's receipt of sessions with a practitioner of the family constellations approach (this model is explained and discussed in Chapter 6) in the hope that it could be a helpful adjunct to our work together. However, the anxiety involved in her planning and managing the journey to and from London for the consultation overshadowed the whole experience for her. I believe the work with her family constellation allowed a slight enhancement in her sense of inner coherence and our therapeutic under-standing and engagement with her process, but again, it didn't provide the level of support and amelioration of her issues for which we both hoped.

DBR

Indicative of her gradual and modest progress through our work together and as a successor to work with her inner parts, in recent years, Angela was able, for a while, to engage with her process and history with DBR. Through these sessions, the themes explored, within our dialogue and the other approaches mentioned, she gained new insights and a breakthrough, of her experiencing an easing of tension and somatic pain by the end of each session. We attended to:

• Angela's terror of sudden, imminent death, with some enhanced clarity of the early sense-memory of something terrible being about to be done to her.
• Her fear of her mother and the drive to please and soothe her. This arose through the exploration of her relationship with her collection of cuddly toys.

By the end of each session, her fear and sensations, including feelings of 'electric shock' and stomach pains, eased enough for her to reflect and be encouraged to con-tinue in our next meeting (while disclosing her apprehension about acknowledging such progress magically causing a later adverse reaction). To provide additional sup-port, I invited her to contact me at any time following a DBR session if she needed to.

However, we had to pause our work with DBR: A client Angela had worked with for 20 years died of cancer, further heightening her fear of death and memories of her mother. This coincided with Angela being overwhelmed and incapacitated by episodes of vertigo and a traumatic consultation with a specialist concerning the issue. Whilst no adverse reaction had occurred during or after DBR sessions, she felt too frightened to continue, fearing the vertigo might be activated and return. Thus, we returned to our more simple dialogic sessions for the process of expres-sion, release, holding and witnessing for her.

Reflections

I have understood Angela's all-consuming terror to be paradoxically a self-protective veiling of specific terrors lodged in her soul and body. This hypothesis resonates with her. As mentioned above, Angela and I (along with the therapist who preceded me) have touched early shadowy and somatic memories of something being or about to be done to her as she lay in bed, convinced she was about to die. However, despite her courage and several different approaches, she has not been able to sustain explorations about this.

Over the years, we have worked together, Angela's slow healing, which commenced with her second therapist, has continued. However, she reminds me of her fear of acknowledging progress when I make such observations as:

- The gargoyles are no longer dominant as images in her consciousness, and her presence is more robust and integrated in her narration and dialogues with me.
- During sessions, she doesn't move toward or into the dark or white rooms.
- Her weight is at an acceptable level.
- Angela allows herself to heat her home in the winter.
- She doesn't have the compulsion to cut herself.
- Suicidal ideation is no longer present in her.

While struggling with whether to resume DBR, Angela shared a story with me about one of her clients whom she has worked with for 17 years. This person, who has also lived with lifelong, debilitating trauma, has recently become able to choose a new, active, fulfilling way of life. Angela lamented that such a capacity still seems unavailable to her, but the significance of this reflection impacted me. Through the expressive proximity of this story to her own, I sensed the potential for such a change present within Angela, manifesting in her faithful holding of her client's healing and movement towards freedom and triumph.

Throughout my work with Angela, I have been profoundly impacted by the depth of her suffering, and at times, felt a sense of desperation and failure paralleling her feelings. I have explored with supervisors for each of the modalities to which I have referred, alongside general supervision, for my practice of gestalt relational psychotherapy. I trust that, on investigation, imperfections will be detected in my use of these approaches. However, my self-examination and self-criticism turn to the occasions in response to her terror and desperation for remedy, where I failed to hold the relationship with the necessary level of inclusion, humility and respect for her soul's journey.

She has told me many times (notwithstanding her wish for me to magically make things better, for her youth to be renewed and to have her life again) that through speaking with me, there is at least the knowledge that one person has heard that with which she has lived and lives. In those moments to which I have just referred, I failed her by ruminating about how I should and could provide more than witnessing and companionship and thus distanced myself from the pain our relationship invoked in me. In those moments, with a combination of self-judgement and self-inflation, I overlooked the full significance of her sharing. From a Gestalt perspective, in the cycles of experience with Angela, I interrupted contact and an I-Thou attitude through confluence with her desperation and activation of introjects from my mother's expectations of me, which paralleled the expectations of Angela's mother.

Sensing my standing alongside the therapists who preceded me (except for the first abusive clinician), for each of whom Angela expresses gratitude, I am reminded of the importance of humility and a therapist's respect for hope and hopelessness. To neither flinch from nor abandon either, with a commitment to be of service as a witness and companion in the expression of horrors commonly deemed to be unspeakable and denied from consciousness.

We continue our close, deepening collaboration, strengthened by my acknowledging her through sharing (albeit less severe) parallels from my process and history. Angela is immensely moved by and committed to the publication of this case study as a documented record and validation of her personal truth and lonely journey. Almost as powerful is her terror of retribution *via* some catastrophic misfortune, in alignment with the weight of suffering she has been fated to carry all her life.

Of Angela and her family, I think of these lines from Davoine and Gaudilliere:

> The destruction…of the guarantees of speech, and the destruction of all reference points, leave the subject who is confronted with them in a state of total estrangement, of absolute aloneness…This alienation from the world is transmitted to whichever of the person's descendants [who] try…to communicate and demonstrate the deafening screams that were left in a state of suspension.
>
> (2004, p. xxviii)

This theme will be present in the next chapter concerning the transgenerational dimension.

References

Davoine, F. & Gaudilliere, G.M. (2004) *History Beyond Trauma.* New York: Other Press.

Forgash, C. & Copeley, M. (Editors, 2008) *Healing the Heart of Trauma and Dissociation with EMDR and Ego State Therapy.* New York: Springer.

Kalsched, D. (2013) *Trauma and the Soul: A Psycho-spiritual Approach to Human Development and Its Interruption.* London & New York: Routledge.

Schwartz, R.C. & Sweezy, M (2020) *Internal Family Systems Therapy*, Second Edition. New York & London: Guildford Press.

Shapiro, F. (2001) *Eye Movement Desensitization and Reprocessing: Basic Principles, Protocols, and Procedures*, Second Edition. New York: Guildford.

Van der Hart, O., Nijenhuis, E.R.S. & Steele, K. (2006) *The Haunted Self: Structural Dissociation and the Treatment of Chronic Traumatization.* London & New York: Norton.

Watkins, J.G. & Watkins, H.H. (1997) *Ego States: Theory and Therapy.* London & New York: Norton.

Chapter 6

The Transgenerational Dimension

As I compose this chapter, present in my consciousness are the catastrophes of violence and suffering taking place around the world, each with individual, familial, and collective threads of grief, entangled loyalties, love, and hate. I believe, with attention to the wounds and systemic entanglements of our histories, a healing can occur for us to be freed from cycles of grief, alienation and suffering that are globally manifest and mirrored back to us.

It is an obvious truth, curiously necessary to repeat in a book concerned with psychotherapy, that the history of past generations influences our consciousness and relationship to self and life. This understanding is held naturally by cultures of the world. For example, Judy Atkinson, describing Aboriginal worldviews, writes:

> *...there is recognition of those who have gone before and their contribution to the whole of who we are, of the connections and communications between people down the generations, between people and country, and between the corporeal and non-corporeal world...*

> (2002, p. 29)

A little later in the text, Atkinson shares with us an important insight concerning the collective and transgenerational trauma of Aboriginal people, which she substantiates within her book:

> *...These inter-relationships must be considered in any developing understanding of the traumatic effects of colonialism where irrevocable intrusion has occurred, and continues to occur, into the soul and fabric of the relationships that people had with each other and their country.*

> (2002, p. 30)

In the conduct of psychotherapy and counselling, attention to clients' ancestral histories is not routinely provided within the initial assessment process or included within its framework. However, I believe for psychotherapy to be a balanced and

DOI: 10.4324/9781003456438-7

inclusive process, the transgenerational dimension needs to be integrated within its theory and practice, with the degree of attention to it necessarily varying according to the background and therapeutic needs of the person (as manifested in their cycles of experiencing within sessions). So, in some cases, the transgenerational will be in the foreground of therapy, and in others, it may be a more subtle but still significant presence. I have sought to demonstrate this in the work with clients presented in this book.

When I commence work with a client, alongside information commonly sought at the start of therapy, I enquire about their ancestry and significant events, traumas and issues that have occurred in the past few generations. These include war, genocide, expulsion and immigration, murder, child deaths, suicide, abuse and the exclusion of family members. I consider gathering and exploring such information within our initial conversations an essential aspect of my preparation for therapeutic work with a client. This is because our orientation to self, others and life is affected by the legacies of previous generations. I understand this inheritance to be carried and transmitted within early, formative relational contact and the interactive and transpersonal fields of our families and communities.

At the end of the previous chapter, I provided a quote from Davoine and Gaudilliere concerning their understanding of the transgenerational transmission of trauma. These words from their chapter in Laub and Hamburger's 'Psychoanalysis and Holocaust Testimony: Unwanted Memories of Social Trauma' (2017) also evoke the potency of that which has been ignored or denied for it to later irrupt *via* transgenerational entanglements and manifest in the lives of people in succeeding generations: 'Madness is a war against denial and perverted social links, waged in order to restore the given word and explore historical truths...' (p. 98).

To those words from Davoine and Gaudilliere, Caruth's (1995) use of the concept of latency provides a complimentary clarification concerning the nature of trauma and its later, transgenerational expression: '...in trauma the greatest confrontation with reality may also occur as an absolute numbing to it, that immediacy, paradoxically enough, may take the form of belatedness' (p. 6).

And, in alignment with the views of the writers above, Laub and Hamburger, in the Introduction to their book, help us to appreciate some of the conditions for the latency and expression with 'immediacy' and 'belatedness' of profoundly shocking individual and collective suffering, which can affect subsequent generations: –

> Both in the event and memory of the Holocaust, there was a breakdown of intrapersonal and interpersonal communication. To address the catastrophe, defensive processes were set in motion side by side with patches of erasure or non-recognition of the experience. What emerged were 'shards of memory' – fragments at once of shattered experience and of the defensive operations attempting to contain them. These found their way into fragmented narratives re-enactments, re-experiencing, transference, and most strikingly, an abundance of countertransference phenomena.
>
> (2017, pp. 4–5)

Transgenerational Trauma and Therapy: The Transgenerational Atmosphere (2020) by Bako and Zana complements the work of the writers cited above. It is an analysis of the intrapsychic, relational and systemic dynamics within traumatised families, through which offspring come to carry and psychologically manifest symptomatic horrors from the past. Based upon work with Holocaust survivors and the succeeding generations, the writers conceptualise this as taking place through a 'transgenerational atmosphere' and collective 'we-experience' (2020), which hold the traumas of previous generations. Within such a domain, from which there is limited contact and trust in the contemporary environment, a process is formed that catalyses the symptomatic experience of the effects of traumas from the past.

The work of the authors I have cited is helpful for understanding a wide range of transgenerational processes that occur within families and communities. These are belated manifestations concerning occurrences such as tragic deaths, sexual abuse or a rupture within the family, which shock the collective soul of a group but have been discounted and denied full expression. The family constellation approach, which I explore and discuss a little later in this chapter, has made an important contribution to the understanding and addressing of these issues.

I also note, from the realm of the physical sciences, epigenetic research confirms the possibility of intergenerational transmission of both the adverse effects of trauma and the passing down of personal resilience (Bowers & Yehuda, 2020), with encouraging findings concerning the efficacy of psychotherapy in modifying epigenetic conditioning (Yehuda et al., 2013).

The Transgenerational as an Influence upon All Our Lives

By turning to face and process the transgenerational endowment from my family history, which I described in Chapter 1, I gained an understanding of how the ancestral past can be a significant force in our lives. I am grateful to Ken Evans for compassionately challenging me during my psychotherapy training in the early 1990s to face how two millennia of anti-Jewish hate, culminating in the Holocaust, has affected me. Such a psychotherapeutic perspective needs to include the enduring impact upon current generations of the full range of collective catastrophes such as the slave trade, colonialism, war and the current ongoing human tragedies occurring in Ukraine and Israel/Palestine. Sadly, the consequent immense suffering from such events that span our world is one of the reasons why the transgenerational dimension is an unending requirement for the theory and practice of psychotherapy.

Over years of clinical work, study and reflection, I have come to appreciate the transgenerational as an influence in our lives, of which mass tragedies are only the more shocking examples. Understanding the processes involved in the latency and expression of such events enables an extension of our knowledge for a general appreciation of how issues stemming from our ancestry affect our consciousness, self and life.

When ancestral issues and events which shock a family or community have not been allowed expression and integration within the individual and collective soul, their later manifestation is a call for therapeutic attention. Thus, it is vital to hold a transgenerational perspective to support a client with such issues and for us to explore them together.

Family Constellations: A Soulful, Systemic Approach to the Transgenerational

In conversation with Sonu Shamdasani in 'Lament of the Dead: Psychology after Jung's The Red Book' (2013), James Hillman said, '...the biggest of all collective problems...is the suppression of the dead. Not hearing the voices of history' (p. 151). I take these words as necessary guidance concerning the implications of a failure to identify historical legacies from events which shock and affect the well-being of a family system and culture, such as war, genocide, forced migration, murder, child deaths and suicide. This is because when there is such 'suppression', a symptomatic expression of history *via* problems such as dysfunctional relating, self-harm, terror, shame and guilt will not be adequately addressed.

It is in alignment with such understanding that the family constellation approach, developed by Bert Hellinger and his colleagues ('Love's Hidden Symmetry', Hellinger, Weber & Beaumont, 1998), addresses the systemic and transpersonal nature of transmissions from the past. I find the model's concept of 'entanglement' helpful in understanding a person's or a group's issues and difficulties. It avoids pathologising individuals or groups and instead considers the broader context of their situation. Beaumont (2012) writes that rather than using terms such as 'neurosis or character', he prefers:

> ...the word 'entanglement' because it also includes our social and historical connections and obligations. Entanglements keep us from developing our potential for good and leave us at the mercy of the negative effects of the past.
>
> (p. 29).

The family constellations model engages with the collective unconscious and interactive field I referred to Chapter 4 to uncover discounted, hidden or suppressed ancestral issues affecting contemporary individual and collective fields of experience. Through professional and personal experience, I learned that working with the constellation of a family system can identify ways we carry significant unconscious identifications to and entanglements with people who suffered, were lost or excluded from the family in previous generations. The approach works by uncovering such patterns of systemic and transgenerational disturbance towards liberating a person living with such issues.

I value this way of looking at transgenerational experiencing as aiding:

- The uncovering, expression and resolution of disturbing issues and hidden entanglements for the re-balancing and the unfolding of our lives.

- Connection with, honouring and enrichment from our ancestral lines.
- Our availability for contact and fulfilment in our lives.
- Support for our personal journey and freedom from those beliefs held within our family and culture that restrict our self-realisation.

These matters are central in the descriptions of my work, which I offer in the next chapter and within this book.

Blind and Enlightened Love

The family constellation model holds an understanding that when a person or persons have been lost in extreme circumstances or excluded, it disturbs the soul of a family. If not expressed, honoured and integrated within the consciousness of the system, it will reverberate through the generations with consequences. One of these can be descendants living through 'blind love' (Schneider, 2007) about those lost or excluded. Blind love is defined as an orientation in which the person's needs are overridden in deferent self-sacrifice to the suffering of parents, other members of the family and ancestors. It can manifest with self-sabotaging behaviours, risky life-threatening actions and suicide.

Through family constellation work, identifying issues and entanglements can release a person from blind love for them to go forward with 'enlightened love' (Schneider, 2007). Enlightened love involves remembering and honouring those who suffered, were lost and/or excluded, with a forward flow of heart energy, to live well, with reverence for the gift of life. In this way, liberation can be found from tormenting, burdening identifications, trauma, guilt and concomitant self-defeating ways of life, allowing space and energy for the opening to a greater appetite for life and living. It is illustrated in one of the case studies in the next chapter concerning Michael and the suffering of his parents in the Second World War.

The perspective of the family constellation model is consistent with Davoine and Gaudilliere's findings from their work with people diagnosed as insane, with madness being the expression of individual and collective traumas which haven't been signified, expressed and acknowledged (2004). For example, Schneider writes:

> Family constellations go beyond the concept of a purely personal experience of trauma to include trauma that has been the fate of others, primarily those we are bound to in empathy and blind love and in a kind of unconscious attempt to balance and compensate. This, too, extends beyond the limits of present time and space.
>
> (2007, p. 32)

Emphasising the transpersonal depth of this work, Daan van Kampenhout has created an approach which is a synthesis of the family constellation model with shamanism, and in 'The Tears of the Ancestors' (2008), he describes and explores the individual soul, 'tribal soul' and the 'universal soul' with respect to transgenerational trauma. Such consideration of the transpersonal dimension supports an inclusive understanding of issues carried and expressed through a person. It is present within the work I share in this book, such as with Lily, in the next chapter.

Outline of a Family Constellation Workshop

My approach includes an adaptation and integration of this model within my one-to-one work rather than workshops, about which I write later in the next chapter. However, to elucidate the principles of the model and my application of them, I will here provide a brief description of the process of a family constellation workshop.

Family constellations work through the direct experience of the issue holder, representatives for members of the family system and the facilitator: 'Constellations basically look at two questions. Firstly, what entangles one family member in the fate of another and what might resolve this entanglement? Secondly, what is needed to support a free flow of love?' (Schneider, 2007, p. 32).

The process commences with the issue holder sitting next to the facilitator to be asked to share the 'burning issue' and 'heart's desire' for which they seek help. It is vital that they hold sufficient energy concerning this matter for the constellation to be configured and unfold. Following this initial conversation, the facilitator will invite the issue holder to choose, one by one, people from the group to represent members of their family, other relevant people and themselves. The issue holder will then intuitively guide each representative to their initial position within the constellation.

Members of the group chosen to be representatives act in the service of the issue holder's family system. The information in thoughts, feelings and movements which emerge through them is often extraordinary. Different explanations have been offered for this remarkable phenomenon, including Rupert Sheldrake's theory of 'morphic fields' (Sheldrake, 2011) and Vivian Broughton's use of concepts concerning unconscious processes such as transference, projection and projective identification (2013). More broadly, for everyone involved in this work, Hunter Beaumont (2023), in an online interview with Tanja Meyburgh, eloquently describes the profound challenge and significance of the endeavour of attunement with the depth within us and the collective field, which enables family constellation work to be beneficial.

Commonly, a constellation will commence with a few people, such as the father, mother and issue holder, with more representatives added as the work progresses. An unfolding exploration within the family system will then take place from the information manifested and expressed through the representatives, the reactions from the issue holder and the attuned guidance of the facilitator. Through this process, systemic entanglements between the issue holder and other members of the family system can be uncovered and addressed, aiding their connection with self, personal needs and heart's desires: enlightened love. The work may involve the voicing of deeply held feelings of loss and grief and suggested sentences of gratitude, bows and blessings towards parents and ancestors. Where traumatised patterns stretch back several generations, a long line of representatives for ancestral mothers and fathers may be asked to stand behind the issue holder to enable their feeling, sensing and connection with ancestral support, which predates the trauma and entanglement. However, sometimes, the history of entangled trauma and suffering goes back so many generations that adding unnamed representatives for the timeless and transpersonal is necessary for connection and to bring holding and support for the issue holder and current generation (Beaumont, 2012, p. 43).

In these ways, family constellations can facilitate resolutions which support the flow of love within the family soul and the freedom of the issue holder to be present in their contemporary reality and self, rather than having their self and life derailed by traumas from the past. Family constellation workshops are a potentially powerful way of attending to transgenerational issues held within the individual and collective unconscious, which have manifested to disturb and distort our lives. Attunement, contact and exploration of the depth are the core factors for the effectiveness of such work, and I strive to support these in my practice of one-to-one psychotherapy.

Family Constellations: A Reservation – My Approach

I have reservations about the capacity for family constellation workshops to be consistently beneficial and effective. As Beaumont articulated in the interview I have cited, the process depends upon a considerable level of commitment and attunement from all involved: the issue holder, representatives, and, crucially, the facilitator's discerning guidance of the proceedings. I also have concerns about the possibility of the process being contaminated by the projection and attribution of attitudes and personal material held by representatives onto the issue, issue holder and the family system. Family constellations require facilitation with an extraordinarily high level of attunement, skill and strength to work with the issue holder, representatives and the manifesting soul-field in a manner which enables accurate and effective attention in the service of the issue holder and their family. In the hands of a strong, experienced and wise practitioner such as Beaumont, a family constellation can be a profoundly enlightening and helpful experience.

In 2004, I completed a two-year training in this approach with the Hellinger Institute of Britain. Still, I understood that I didn't yet have access to the inner strength required to fulfil the responsibilities of a facilitator in family constellation workshops. So, I committed myself to applying learning from this model within my practice of psychotherapy with individuals. Integral to my exploration with clients through their cycles of experience is a reverence for the presence and expressions from the mysterious depths of our being, as manifested in constellation workshops.

I have found that through attuned, therapeutic dialogue, including sensing, seeing and imaginal conversing with parents, family members and ancestors, we can explore systemic and transgenerational issues and legacies a client has lived with. In such work involving the struggles, suffering and traumas of previous generations, I may offer sentences and imaginal experiments for the client to use or say (with modification at their discretion) to a family member or members for soulful connection and resolution of an entanglement. Alternatively, I might suggest their noticing insights which have arisen and allow understanding of, and compassion for their ancestors and themself concerning burdens and restrictions with which they have been living. Being with clients in their cycles of experience in these ways is integral to the process, as expression and integration occur for that which had been unseen and dissociated from the collective and individual soul. This supports the client's uncovering, realisation and journey of self in this life, which were discussed in earlier chapters.

To enhance the process, I may offer exercises with visualisation, Playmobil figures or floor tiles to facilitate and work with a family constellation:

Visualisation: As in my description in Chapter 4 concerning work in the imaginal dimension, I will ask a client to look at their place in relation to parents, family members and other people with whom issues are connected; to work with their direct experience through this inner sight, felt sense and emotions.

Playmobil Figures: Using Playmobil figures as representatives for family members is another way of enacting the constellating process. Having decided on the issue to be explored, I will ask my client to choose a Playmobil figure for each person to be included in the constellation. I suggest they take a few slow, deep breaths and sense their body being held by the chair and feet by the floor. I then ask them to allow feelings (if the client is of a spiritual disposition, I will say 'soul') to intuitively guide their hand to move and place each figure individually. When the constellation has been set up, I will ask my client to look and report upon their experience of seeing the symbolic depiction of the family system and relationships, holding the chosen issue lightly. We will then proceed with exploring the constellation, as in a workshop *via* my facilitation. I ask my client to place a finger on top of each figure to sense and receive feelings and information that come from the person represented, with movements of experimental sentences to and between the figures. As the work unfolds, we may add figures representing other people or aspects of the person's existential desires and dilemmas.

As in a constellation workshop, it is important that this work is carried out with respect and an attitude of service to the whole family. This encourages attunement and access to the depth and the processing of the systemic factors that have underlain the client's issue.

Floor tiles: I use this approach with clients who have a good level of inner support and stability and can manage the stress and intrapsychic challenges it can induce because of the embodied connections and shifts to and from different people represented in the constellation.

I will ask my client to place a floor tile for each person to be included at the beginning of this work with the constellation. Our exploration will again follow the workshop process, with the client standing on the tiles to tune into and speak as each person represented by a floor tile. As always, this must be held and conducted with respect and care for the client and the souls being represented. Given the power and challenge of this way of activating the constellating process, the pace of work must be carefully calibrated *via* attunement to the client and the field of soul being touched by us.

Childhood and Our Parents within Soul-Based Systemic Work

A transgenerational attitude towards childhood experiences and our relationships with parents and primary care providers can support healing and personal unfolding. In 'Towards a Spiritual Psychotherapy' (2012), Beaumont distinguishes between our 'essential' parent who loves us profoundly, and our 'entangled' parent. The latter's ways, which were unhelpful (*e.g.* oppressive, shaming and negligent) for us as children, were expressions of the burdens they have carried from entanglements, trauma and existential struggles. In our relationships with them, we will have made creative adjustments in our beliefs and behaviour and, in time, come to hold these as fixed gestalts of conformity, avoidance and/or rebellion. Beaumont suggests we can be liberated and enriched through opening to awareness of and connection with the essence of our parents, beneath their persona and the destructive aspects of their entangled parenting of us. A reverence for our parents' essence affirms our connection with the depth of being.

Beaumont describes how 'Feelings of justified resentment' against our family can leave us 'dependent and incomplete' (2012, pp. 8–9). He counsels that in relationships with our parents, 'When we are able to remember our father's essence we do better, our children do better and our father does better' (2012, p. 33), and a 'soul movement towards our mother's essence can succeed because we are reaching out to the potential behind our entangled mother' (2012, p. 59). This is illustrated in the case study in the next chapter concerning my work with Michael. I respect this aspect of Lily's holding of her complex relationship with her mother, which I described in Chapter 5, and that with her father in Chapter 7.

The above understanding does not imply a discounting of the psychological injuries and deficits we carry from childhood and the importance of feeling, expressing and healing from them. However, when we are ready to explore in the way Beaumont suggests, we can open to the love and space for acceptance of essence, within and between us. In this way, we may find resolution of developmental and transgenerational trauma and become more mature as people, with freedom from the confines of object relations and dynamics within our family system. In a vignette in Chapter 8, concerning my work with Sabine, we see her movement towards clarity concerning the holding, protective, affirming legacy she carries from her father, with an easing of both her experience of rejection and patterns of reactive action, borne of transgenerational trauma.

In the next chapter, I offer five examples of my work with the transgenerational dimension.

References

Atkinson, J. (2002) *Trauma Trails, Recreating Song Lines: The Transgenerational Effects of Trauma in Indigenous Australia.* Victoria: Spinifex.

Bako, T. & Zana, K. (2020) *Transgenerational Trauma and Therapy: The Transgenerational Atmosphere.* Abingdon, Oxon: Routledge.

Beaumont, H. & Meyburgh, T. (2023) *Our Tribute to Hunter Beaumont*. Available at: https://realacademy.net/#tribute (Accessed: 26 August 2024).

Beaumont, H. (2012) *Toward a Spiritual Psychotherapy: Soul as a Dimension of Experience*. Berkeley, CA: North Atlantic Books.

Bowers, M.E. & Yehuda, R. (2020) *Intergenerational transmission of Stress Vulnerability and resilience*. New York: Icahn School of Medicine at Mount Sinai.

Broughton, V. (2013) Gestalt, trauma, constellations. In: *British Gestalt Journal* 2013, Vol 22, No. 2, pp. 14–24.

Caruth, C. (1995, Editor) *Introduction: Trauma: Explorations in Memory*. Baltimore, MD & London: The John Hopkins University Press.

Davoine, F. & Gaudilliere, G.M. (2017) The psychoanalysis of psychosis at the crossroads of individual stories and of history. In *Psychoanalysis and Holocaust Testimony: Unwanted Memories of Social Trauma*. Laub, D. & Hamburger, A. (Editors). London & New York: Relational Book Series, Routledge, pp. 92–103.

Davoine, F. & Gaudilliere, G.M. (2004) *History Beyond Trauma*. New York: Other Press.

Hellinger, B. with Weber, G. & Beaumont, H. (1998) *Love's Hidden Symmetry. What Makes Love Work in Relationships*. Phoenix, AZ: Zeig, Tucker & Co.

Hillman, J. & Shamdasani, S. (2013) *Lament of the Dead: Psychology after Jung's Red Book*. New York: Norton.

Kampenhout, D.V. (2008) *The Tears of the Ancestors: Victims and Perpetrators in the Tribal Soul*. Phoenix, AZ: Zelig, Tucker & Theison.

Laub, D. & Hamburger, A. (2017, Editors) Introduction to: *Psychoanalysis and Holocaust Testimony: Unwanted Memories of Social Trauma*. London & New York: Relational Book Series, Routledge.

Schneider, J.R. (2007) *Family Constellations: Basic Principles and Procedures*. Heidelberg: Carl-Auer.

Sheldrake, R. (2011) *The Presence of the Past: Morphic Resonance and the Habits of Nature*, Second Edition. London: Icon Books.

Yehuda, R., Daskalakis, N.P., Desarnaud, F., Makotkine, I., Lehrner, A.L., Koch, E., Flory, J.D., Buxbaum, J.D., Meaney, M.J. & Bierer, L.M. (2013). Epigenetic biomarkers as predictors and correlates of symptom improvement following psychotherapy in combat veterans with PTSD. In: *Frontiers in Psychiatry: Molecular Psychiatry* September 2013, Volume 4, Article 118.

Chapter 7

The Transgenerational Dimension in Practice

In the descriptions of my work with clients, I seek to demonstrate my integrative approach to the transgenerational dimension and the self in my psychotherapy practice. Their background, needs and capacity determine the prominence of the transgenerational in the therapeutic process, and I strive to be responsive in meeting them where they are in their ongoing journeys of healing and unfolding. There are transgenerational dynamics present in some of my case studies, which could have been pursued further if it had been appropriate to their figural, emergent needs and the arising gestalts of their process.

I Return to My Work with Lily

Her father is a political refugee from an Eastern European country. He arrived in the UK decades before Lily's birth, having found himself in peril and needing to escape. For their safety, he left his family without notice. When he was safely established in the UK, letters were exchanged between them, but it was ten years before he visited to meet with them again. From her early childhood, Lily experienced her father as overbearing and preoccupied with communicating his own specialness and that of her aunt, his sister. As a consequence, Lily had a complicated and troubled relationship with her father, feeling both an aversion to contact with him and a yearning for his adoring fatherly gaze.

When she was two years old, her father had a breakdown, a manifestation of the trauma he carries. It was a precipitating factor in his separation from her mother. He told Lily of an episode at a chess tournament when he took shelter under the table, then returned home, lay on the floor and asked Lily's mother to call for help. Lily was playing upstairs in her bedroom whilst this occurred.

In the context of our work together, the following two pieces of work were helpful in Lily's progress towards release from entanglement with her father's issues. They allowed her to become more confident and relaxed with him and soulfully connected with her Eastern European family and ancestors.

- I asked Lily to bring her father to her mind's eye, face him, notice the direction and quality of his gaze and her disposition and feelings towards him. Lily saw

DOI: 10.4324/9781003456438-8

her father look away and felt a familiar sense of disappointment and deflation. We proceeded to work, with a slow, gentle exchange of poignant contact between them, using honouring and freeing sentences. Lily thanked him for her life, and with a symbolic forward movement of her arms, she respectfully passed back to him the traumas from his life that had impinged upon her own experience of self. The exercise culminated in her experiencing his affirming gaze and blessing.

- During a session involving the exploration of a nightmare in which Lily and her husband were attacked, we sensed a connection with the tumultuous family history in Eastern Europe. We set up a constellation, using Playmobil figures to represent her Eastern European family and her father. Through touching the figures, sensing her connection with them and exchanging sentences of acknowledgement and respect, she felt seen and accepted by them for herself in her dual heritage. It was a liberating experience, which helped Lily feel connected with them, free of her father's entanglement.

Rose

Rose is an accomplished consultant and writer, who contacted me, explaining she was:

> …looking for help with transgenerational trauma… Last week a close friend who is also a trained counsellor named a feeling I didn't previously have a name for as "transgenerational trauma" which made some things begin to fall into place. Both of my grandfathers survived world wars, the first came back from WWI minus a foot, the second came back from WWII physically intact but emotionally battered, I suspect they both had PTSD, and this has effects on me and on my family that I would like to understand.

In the early sessions, Rose shared with me more information concerning the systemic and transgenerational issues that affected her early years of life. She told me that from the age of 6, she felt she was needed as a carer to her parents. In that same year, her maternal grandmother died, following which her mother suffered from depression, with all her maternal aunts being similarly affected. Rose's father was also in poor health for much of her childhood. She informed me that from an early age, she suffered bullying at school. I, thus, gained a strong sense of Rose's isolation as a child, and her carrying an intense focus upon, and attentiveness for other people. She powerfully conveyed to me a sense of not having been able to really live and enjoy her childhood. During our work together, she would tell me of feeling weight and pressure on her shoulders, pushing her down. When I facilitated Rose's exploration of her experience through visualisation and sensing within the imaginal dimension, she was unable to see, feel or connect with supportive, resourcing figures.

Figure Work

Early in our work together, I invited Rose to choose figures to represent her father, mother and herself. She placed them in a line, with mother and father facing each other, and Rose standing between them. I asked her to notice what went on inside as she looked at this scene. Rose reflected later:

> From the best of my memory, I wasn't facing either parent; they were facing each other, and I was in between them facing outwards. So – and this has only just occurred to me – I had an ear to each parent, which is perhaps more relevant than where my face was pointing.

Key issues carried by her parents, as expressed through the Playmobil figures were:

- Her father's experiences as an evacuee, whilst her grandfather was in a prisoner of war camp.
- Her mother, having left her family of origin to marry Rose's father, felt unable to cope with marriage and parenthood.

The work with these figures provided Rose with a vivid representation of being born to two people weighed down by history who were not ready to be parents, and her experience of being pulled by love to help each of them. This brought to the foreground an awareness that she 'couldn't be a child and had to be an adult' and related to her somatic experiencing of 'weight' and 'pressure', of which she spoke many times in our work together. Rose said she found the session 'illuminating'. I believe it was pivotal in the development of our work together.

When we met the following week, Rose said the session had been freeing. She appeared changed; her presence was stronger. There were long, rich silences as we sat together, which I felt were resonating deep contact. I sensed space had opened within her, between and from the introjects: and the weight and pressure she carried. This was reflected in her relaxed reflections and wishes, which had flowed from the previous sessions. I sensed a holiness in the room, which remained after she had left and to which I bowed.

From this session onwards our work progressed, with an integration within our therapeutic dialogue of Gestalt two-chair work to explore self-parts within Rose's psyche.

Four significant parts which Rose identified, named and explored during our work together were:

- The manager, who had a driven attitude and was focussed on tasks.
- The sergeant-major, a holding, supportive figure for her.
- A young child, withdrawn in shadow, frightened by and ashamed of her feelings.
- Another young child with a more vivid, robust image, who faced away, wanting to be and play, by herself.

As our work progressed, Rose identified a desire 'to be whole' and accept all parts of herself and her feelings. She had dreams of babies and pregnancy, which I understood to be an expression of her opening towards self-acceptance and realisation.

In the course of research and conversations with friends, Rose became progressively confident that she was neurodiverse – autistic. As this became clearer to her, her acceptance of self and peaceful experiencing increased. This period was also marked with anxiety regarding the possibility that the formal assessment might not concur with her sensing and understanding of herself. When her self-diagnosis was confirmed, Rose felt deep relief and a profound movement towards acceptance of both herself and others. She noticed a falling away from the overriding feeling of obligation in response to other peoples' expectations, wishes and needs, which had dominated her life since infancy.

Reflecting upon her experiences of bullying, she felt an equanimity, which included an understanding of those who treated her in such intolerant and unkind ways as being the consequence of their ignorance of her being autistic. She felt at one with her way of being 'whole', the sense and feeling she had yearned for. She reported enhanced love and acceptance of her partner.

On a perceptual level, Rose noticed how colours appeared brighter and more vivid. Initially, she wondered if this change in her life was a 'blip'. As the weeks passed, her new orientation remained stable, settled and evident in all aspects of her life. Her newfound self-acceptance and equanimity have been enduring.

During the concluding sessions of our work together, Rose emphasised that my acceptance of her had been an essential aspect of the therapeutic experience. I believe that attending to transgenerational entanglements, early formative experiences and different parts of her psyche helped her open up to her wholeness and unique qualities as a human being, which the diagnosis of being neurodiverse formally confirmed for her. Please read Rose's reflections in the appendix to this book.

Catherine

My work with Catherine involved my facilitating her exploration of her relationship with herself and others, which was significantly supported by insights concerning her place within the family system and its history. Through attunement with her cycles of experiencing, I sought to hold a therapeutic balance of attendance to her current life issues and the impact upon these of systemic and transgenerational processes.

Catherine is a professional woman in her 50s who had been troubled since childhood by inhibiting self-doubt, feelings of toxic shame and difficulty in making decisions.

In her engagement with me, she conveyed a self-dismissive attitude in response to my enquiring about her wishes and needs. The issue, figural from the start of our work together, was a tortuous process with an ex-partner.

She provided me with information which was indicative of systemic and transgenerational entanglements:

- Her father was conceived out of wedlock, with his mother stating he was born prematurely due to her feelings of shame. He lived with a generalised experience of self-doubt and shame, which he expressed in poems, some of which Catherine shared with me; she felt much in common with his orientation to self and life.

- Catherine's maternal grandfather was a wounded survivor of the First World War battle of Passchendaele, in which hundreds of thousands of people from both sides were killed. He lived with survivor guilt, which was compounded by his receiving a white feather in a cafe.
- Her mother's elder sister died at birth.
- When Catherine was 22 months old, her mother gave birth to twins, a boy and a girl, both born with cerebral palsy. Her sister died two days after birth. Catherine also has an older sister and another younger brother.

In her first session, Catherine told me that from early in her memory, her mother had voiced an assumption, a conceit, of knowing her from the inside when, in fact, she felt painfully unseen – those moments held a deep significance for Catherine because they were representative of the aspect of her childhood within which she experienced feeling deeply alone, with a lack of attention to, or affirmation of her developing self.

Catherine described her difficulty in asserting and holding boundaries with her ex-partner, who continued to refuse the ending of the relationship several years earlier. When in alternating aggressive and distressed tones, she sought to assert the continuance of the relationship and manipulate her towards that target, Catherine experienced powerful, constricting reactions of guilt and fear. Like her mother, the ex-partner held a presumptuous and condescending attitude to Catherine's needs, feelings and wishes. This was a tortuous process for Catherine, which dominated and paralysed her thoughts and feelings and affected an obscuring of, and lack of attention to her needs.

Catherine's process with her ex-partner was representative of the way she related to herself and other people, and it was an opportunity for exploration and self-realisation. In alignment with her mother's attitude towards her, Catherine was restricted in her engagement with self. I thought the use of the family constellation model in the exploration of her familial relationships could be helpful and facilitated Catherine in her visualising of her parents, siblings and herself.

In the visualisation, she saw herself standing on the perimeter of the family constellation, looking inwards from a place of isolation towards other family members. This was a powerful depiction of her childhood experience, in being distant from contact and the nurturing she needed. Catherine looked with care and deference to the traumas of her mother and her disabled, troubled brother, whilst being inhabited by shame and self-doubt – that which had blighted her father's life.

By seeing the systemic roots of the discounting and suppression of her needs, Catherine experienced the arising of a freeing self-awareness. As a result, the concept she had held of herself and her obligations were loosened, allowing her to connect more with her needs and have greater access to her feelings and heart's desires. I held in my heart and mind what had been revealed in the visualised family constellation, reflecting this to Catherine to support her towards a growing freedom of self.

She became progressively assertive with her ex-partner and, in time, was able to end contact with her, and I witnessed space for and access to her needs and wishes open within her as she formed a new, nourishing relationship with an empathic and caring woman.

Bill

Bill is a professional man in his thirties who has lived with a lack of confidence and energy towards aspects of his personal life that are important to him.

He experienced both his parents as lacking interest in him, except for moments of crisis and the pursuit of forms of achievement with which they identified. When faced with the challenge of pursuing a heart's desire, Bill noted that he had a pattern like his father of withdrawal into self-doubt, procrastination and inaction. Bill was also troubled by his father's self-preoccupied, jealous and competitive attitude towards him. This included a significant childhood memory of when his father reacted destructively to Bill's creative excitement in assembling a crystal radio set.

We worked with floor tiles, and as he stood on the place representing his father, we noticed an absence of attention to Bill and, instead, a movement to look behind. I placed another tile where his gaze fell, and as Bill stood there, expressing arising feelings, it became clear that the figure he was representing in that position was his paternal grandfather. His father turning backwards reflected a preoccupation with feelings of loss and resentment for the lack of attention *he* had received as a child.

Bill's paternal grandfather had a life marked by tragedy. His first wife died in childbirth, and their child died, too. He had a second marriage, which was childless and ended in divorce. By the time of his third marriage and the birth of Bill's father, he was in his fifties. What came through, as Bill stood on the tile for his grandfather, was the latter's limited capacity to parent Bill's father because of grief and his advanced age. The exploration unfolded as Bill inhabited and spoke from and between these three positions. This process helped Bill understand his relationship with his father. It allowed relief from feelings of deficiency and shame as he saw that his father's attitude conveyed the reality of an entanglement formed before his birth. The exercise ended with a dialogue between Bill and his father, in which the latter looked at, acknowledged and affirmed his son.

Michael

Background

Michael's father, Henryk, was Polish and born in 1913, the youngest of seven children in an area which at the time was part of the German Empire. Henryk's father was killed in the First World War, and his mother became a war widow and lone parent. From 1918, this area became part of the newly re-established country of Poland.[1]

At the beginning of the Second World War, Henryk's home area was invaded by the German army and remained under its occupation until the end of the war. He lost a brother following the German invasion and joined the Polish resistance. Henryk, along with all the members of his resistance cell, was captured by the Gestapo at Christmas 1942 and, in the following January, was sent to the Stutthof Concentration Camp. Near the end of the war, along with other survivors of Stutthof, he was sent by the Nazis on 'death marches at sea' of barges and floated out into the Baltic Sea ('Stutthof Maritime Evacuations Project', International Holocaust Remembrance Alliance, 2021). Some people were later placed on German ships with the knowledge that they would be bombed by allied planes. Henryk was one of very few who came through this ordeal, and he was received into a displaced persons camp within the sector of Germany controlled by the Western allies. In June 1948, he was received as a refugee by the UK.

Michael's mother, Maria, was Polish and was born in Poland in 1922 and married her first husband in her teens. He was taken to Siberia by the Soviet forces who occupied their part of Poland until 1941. She did not see or hear from him again. During this period, she lost one of her brothers and also feared the loss of her eldest brother. When Nazi Germany broke its pact with the Soviet Union in 1941, its army took occupation of Maria's home area, and she was subsequently taken to Germany as slave labour, never to return home again. In 1944, the Soviet army retook the area, and during this period, Maria's mother and a second brother died.

From 1945 to 1947, Maria lived in a displaced persons camp where, with the help of the Red Cross, she was found by her eldest brother who, as a pilot, had fought in the Polish squadrons of the RAF and was living in the UK. She arrived in the UK in November 1947. Henryk and Maria met and married in the UK. Their first son, Anthony, died after only a few weeks of life, and Michael was born five years later. Henryk died in the 1990s, followed by Maria in the 2000s.

Michael and I commenced our work on Zoom during the second year of the COVID pandemic. He was in his mid-60s, and his appearance on the screen was pale, frail and anxious, through which came a stoic clarity and determination. From those first moments, I was touched by the sincerity and intensity in his sharing of sorrow, fear and the traumatic memories he carried for his parents.

He told me he wanted to reflect upon the current phase of his life, which he grimly called the 'endgame'. Many years earlier, Michael's previous therapy experience had been about managing feelings of guilt in living apart from his elderly, ailing mother concerning her and his expectations of himself. The pandemic had escalated Michael's withdrawal from his social life and artistic activities, following worries about his health and retirement from employment in a social care service.

Michael told me that his parents withheld information concerning aspects of their traumatic histories until his teens, giving him a fabricated story, which protectively excluded disclosure of Henryk's experiences both in Stutthof Concentration Camp and on the maritime death-march. Henryk sought to guide Michael to grow up as an English boy in this land of refuge for him and Maria.

Michael described himself as being 'the light' of his parents' lives, his precious-ness magnified by the horrors through which they had come, followed by the death of their first child. Michael told me they were 'overprotective' of him, this being an effect of their traumas. As he spoke, I was impacted by the ongoing fear and self-expectations that had marked his life, which he poignantly expressed by quot-ing a Beatles lyric concerning the carrying of a burden.

His father and mother argued, sometimes followed by a silence between them which lasted several days. From childhood through to adulthood, Michael found himself, both carrying and being an intermediary to their conflicts, which I under-stood to be expressive of the pain and weight of their suffering and needs. When conflict between his mother and father was less prominent, Michael described the family unit as being an 'intense tripartite' formation, again poignantly conveying to me their being together in the aftermath of the untold, shattering traumas carried by mother and father. The making of simple domestic decisions was often fraught with a collective angst; as if every decision was still one of survival or death. I thought of Zana and Bako's (2020) concepts of the transgenerational atmosphere and we-experience they use to describe the families of survivors. The fact Michael was clearly and deeply affected by the family history, without fully knowing his parents' stories until his teens serve to emphasise the potential power of interper-sonal processes in the transmission of trauma.

Michael attended school with the dedicated support and hopes of his parents for his academic career, and he was a diligent student, faithful to their loving desires for him. While enjoying aspects of the experience, outside school, Michael was iso-lated, lonely and troubled. He obtained a university place at a prestigious Oxbridge college. For Henryk and Maria, having survived the abyss of the Second World War, one can imagine how special it was for them to see their one child welcomed into such a place and quality of life. However, Michael struggled with university life, experiencing it as a severe personal challenge from which he suffered a break-down. His interest in the arts blossomed at university, but his ill-confidence limited his participation in these activities. Returning home following graduation, Michael eventually moved out at 30, with his life remaining closely intertwined with his parents, especially in the care of his mother.

Relationships

Michael's relationship with his mother up to and beyond her death was marked by confluence with her and the traumas she carried. Through Michael's childhood and adolescence, Maria immersed him in anxious, doting-care, through which he was sheltered from developing an independent routine for self and domestic care. This remained an issue concerning such tasks in his daily life, which we would address in the therapy.

Michael grew up with high expectations of attentiveness to and care for his mother. Sometimes, she chided him with phrases such as 'You're just like your father', which were remarkably similar to his father's rebukes ('You're just like your mother').

When Michael commenced therapy with me, he was single and lived alone. Relationships and friendships with women were matters about which he felt failure and guilt and vividly reflective of the process with his mother. He was often drawn to those who needed help and care, towards whom he strained and strived to please, on occasion at the price of his own needs. Michael named some unfulfilled friendships as 'fantasy relationships', which he had hoped would blossom through his dedication to the person's needs, just as he yearned for his mother's relief from grief and full acceptance of him as a person. He had a generalising sense of failing the women in his life and being flawed.

Beginning Our Work

In the early sessions, Michael was steely determined in his pre-planned recounting of his parents' stories and his own. On occasion, he became overwhelmed by feelings of distress, grief and pessimism concerning his health (he had a few issues, none of which were life-threatening), needing to lie down for a while through the process. I was impacted by Michael's intense drive and desperation to tell me of the history, experiences and issues with which he had lived. I appreciated the lonely path he had walked in striving to contain his pain and be of service to others.

I counselled Michael to ease the pace in sharing and disclosing, explaining the therapeutic value of sensing and attuning to the feelings and experience of his body. I taught and guided him through various soothing, grounding exercises, which he found useful. During these first few weeks, I provided extra sessions to support him in managing his feelings through this phase of painful opening to expression and exploration with me. I facilitated an imaginal exercise (of the type I outlined in Chapter 4) for Michael to access support from within, and there arose for him the soothing presence of a squirrel, bringing him relief and an easing of tension. Discovering the ability to experience release and relaxation was encouraging for him.

Before our work together, Michael had sought to manage the force of family tragedy and trauma in his soul with its fear, shame and guilt, through a cognitive, task-focussed perspective. This attitude matched the offerings from concerned friends. Unfortunately, the failure of this approach to provide an amelioration of his suffering reinforced his sense of failure, deficiency and fault.

In Michael's dialogue with me, a crucial element of the therapeutic process was my holding in my awareness and heart: Michael himself, his parents and their individual and collective history. I felt called by the intensity of his pain, self-judgement and self-deprecation to offer a transgenerational framing of the experiences and issues he was disclosing to me. This brought him relief from his crushing inner-experiencing. He frequently reflected upon his apprehension before the start of a session and his finding this to have been unwarranted, as he ended the session more relaxed and less self-critical. I understood this to be an early indication that the sessions were having a healing effect and a source of relief from his toxic shame.

With developing trust, albeit nervous of judgement, Michael shared with me his attraction to suicide and subscription to an organisation concerned with euthanasia and assisted dying. He didn't intend to kill himself at this time, and we discussed supportive activities which could provide holding between sessions, agreeing that he would contact me or another source of support if his feelings became difficult to manage and contain. He consulted his doctor, who prescribed antidepressants and beta blockers.

Michael conveyed to me the presence of contrasting drives towards death and life. The push towards death came from existential despair and the pain of aloneness in living without his parents. Conversely, the commitment and courage he brought to sessions were a powerful expression of his energy for life. In relation to this issue, the twin concepts of blind and enlightened love, explained in Chapter 6, were meaningful to Michael. He saw that joining his parents through premature death was of the former, and alternatively, to live well honoured them, and the life they gave him was an expression of enlightened love. I also explained the distinction between the entangled and essential aspects of parents, concerning the love he held for them and his need to process those aspects of their relationship, which impinged upon his experience of self and life. He bought and read Hunter Beaumont's book, which I cited and discussed in Chapter 6 with respect to this issue. Such understanding would guide our work together. Michael recorded each of his sessions, finding listening to them again helpful and supportive.

In the third month of our work, Michael told me of his enjoying a better week in which he visited a friend. In this way, he affirmed life by breaking out of his social isolation of nearly two years duration, since the start of the COVID pandemic.

The Ukraine War, a Photograph and Cardigan

In her youth, his mother's hometown had been located within the borders of Poland, but it is now part of modern Ukraine, and this made the shocking nature of the Russian invasion personal for him. Around this time, Michael was moved to look again at a photo from the late 1970s of him standing with his father inside Stutthof Concentration Camp. He was surprised to notice that in the picture, he was physically holding his father. This was visual evidence of his support of his father and provided him with a refreshing insight into the balance of their relationship and his value as a son. Michael also reflected sadly that his father had suddenly aged following this, his only return to Poland following the war and their sole visit together.

In the following session, Michael wore a cardigan of his father's, asking me 'Is this healthy?' I encouraged him to explore his feelings. He felt his connection with his father, and then a discordant memory arose of not being trusted to drive the family car because 'You're like your mother'. Michael told me he felt disloyal in sharing such incidents with me. I offered a reframing perspective, suggesting that such sincere exploration serves personal unfolding and freedom of self, and so is an honouring of the gift of life he received from his good and loving parents.

Moving deeper into his feelings, Michael lamented: 'We weren't able to help each other'. This sentence conveyed the heart-felt desire he carried both as a child and an adult, to help his parents with their suffering and an acceptance that it was something he had been unable to do and that neither was able to protect and prevent him from growing up with the fears they carried.

Terror of Medical Procedures

Through our weekly dialogues and explorations, Michael gradually integrated into his self-understanding a transgenerational appreciation of his emotional life rather than deprecating himself as failing and flawed. For example, he conveyed to me existential terror concerning looming but non-life-threatening medical and dental procedures, all of which weighed heavily on him with dread.

He described his attitude, with words poignantly expressive of the traumas carried by his parents, as each medical procedure being akin to a 'battle in a losing war' and the movement towards death. I suggested to Michael, given his parent's experience of extreme violence across all aspects of life under Nazi and Soviet rule, that it was understandable for them to be gravely apprehensive of contact with figures of authority, including medical professionals, and that this fear had been transmitted to him.

Michael came through the medical and dental procedures, finding them less stressful than he had anticipated. I believe this was a healing episode for him; by processing his terror about these events and experiencing them to integrate a distinction between his contemporary reality and the past endured by his parents and family.

Release from Transgenerational Trauma

With respect to Michael's belief that he had failed his parents and his female friends, I understood that the standard by which he had been judging himself was, in effect, the amelioration of another person's suffering. This perspective was a product of his loving entanglement with his parents' experience of apocalypse – the horrors, tragedies and ultimate survival which occurred before he was born. We explored the parallels in his relationships and friendships with women in his life, past and present, and how their suffering activated a transference onto them of his drive to help and meet his mother. In this process, the loving eyes exercise I described in Chapter 4 was helpful, providing compassionate, soothing contact with the anxious and driven part of himself that arose into the foreground in contact with women.

A significant, touching moment for Michael, which he would refer to in future sessions, occurred when I facilitated a visualisation of him facing his parents within his mind's eye. The purpose of this exercise was for soulful exploration outside the confines of his normative beliefs and judgements. In this contact with his parents within the imaginal dimension, there was an affirming of his relationship with them and a lightening of the burden of judgement which had affected his life. He saw love in their faces and felt its depth from and for them. I supported him in his expressions of gratitude and respect for them, to which he sensed a corresponding wish and pleasure from them for him to prosper in his life. In time, he would come to understand his father's expectations, with a modified perspective of Henryk wishing him to honour their history but 'not be crippled by it'.

With the easing of the COVID pandemic, Michael gradually resumed direct social contact, including resuming his artistic activities. As he re-engaged with life, it was lovely to see and sense the change in him. During our work together, a new friendship had been slowly forming for Michael through meetings in city parks with careful social distancing. Jessica, warmly engaged with Michael and his life rather than being hungry for his help and care, which, as previously stated, had been characteristic of many of his contacts with women. From enjoying their time together, Michael explored with me his experience of Jessica's interest, care and acceptance as dormant hopes and feelings began to open in him.

One day, they touched each other with the tips of one finger, and in time, with the receding of the pandemic, their relationship developed. From his smile and the light in his eyes, which had begun to mark the start of many sessions, the expansion of life within him was evident and beautiful to see. He began to progressively share with Jessica more of his own and his family's history whilst still experiencing familiar feelings of shame, being flawed and fears that he might burden and overwhelm her.

However, in time, Michael came to accept that she was keen and able to listen and learn about him. This contact with Jessica became part of his process of healing and personal unfolding, in which he experienced both a growing sense of being alive and a residual feeling of deadness. Also present were self-judgement, harsh demands of himself to 'work harder' and a belief of being 'diseased' – irreparably damaged like his mother. In weekly sessions, through holding, clarifying and processing *via* the transgenerational perspective, there was confirmation of Michael's self and path of individuation, distinct from the family narrative. The use of DBR, with an activating stimulus for these issues verbalised by a desperate 'I've got to work harder to make myself better' and an anchoring orienting tension at the back of his head, provided relief for him to be moved and announce, 'I'm going to let Jessica in… I'm doing well'.

Michael's relationship with Jessica blossomed, his optimism expanded, and as a result new questions began to arise for him. The diminution of pain and despair, and the rise of hope and pleasure, brought him to voice concern about a lifestyle distinct from the transgenerational atmosphere of his family and of relaxing into being a 'lotus eater' – a hedonist. He asked me, 'What is well-being?' in an expression of a deepening consideration concerning the qualities in his life which had been pushed into the background by stoicism in the face of misery.

The Suitcase Which Became a 'Toolbox' for Healing

Michael's attention turned towards the suitcase his mother had purchased in the 1950s. It contained documents and photos related to his parents' lives and his own childhood. It also held a statement left for him by his father concerning his experiences in Stutthof Concentration Camp, on the maritime death marches, and in the displaced persons camp.

Michael had expressed troubled, ambivalent feelings about the suitcase and its contents in earlier sessions. He had thought about destroying most of the material because of its raw, unprocessed weight that lay upon his soul, the unintegrated past within his memory. Now, with Jessica's interest and support, he began to look again, carefully reading and sharing the history and meaning of the contents with her. Aware of Michael's drive and expectations by which he can overwhelm himself, I advised that he monitor his feelings and emotions through this process and take breaks when necessary to ground and reorient himself. This was to support his digestion and processing of the evocations and personal and soulful significance of these artefacts. It was important to avoid reactivating (and reinforcing) transgenerational trauma through a loss of here-now experiencing of self.

Michael received a significant dream with respect to the process of disentanglement from his family history. In the dream, his mother was still alive; a record of her wartime experiences had been written, and he felt angry and ashamed, believing it was his duty to have composed the piece.

We explored the dream through Michael visualising and sensing the dream's cast of people and component parts within his mind's eye. He made calm, imaginal contact with his mother. In the light of conversations concerning his sense of duty to make public information concerning his parents' suffering, I suggested he ask her for permission to share the document with an appropriate archive. She approved, and Michael visualised himself doing so by meeting an archivist and passing on the material. This affected a powerful discharge of tension, with a feeling of relief provided by the realisation that he didn't have to hold onto the horror and that its significance can be conveyed into the world. It was a step in undoing the entanglement with his mother's suffering, which had been carried in the dream. As we reflected together upon this piece of dreamwork, Michael again found helpful the distinction between the entangled behaviour of his mother and her essential quality of love for him, as manifested in this and previous exercises within the imaginal dimension.

The therapeutic process of expression and unburdening was supported through Michael's learning that his worry about sharing with Jessica was unfounded. She was not overwhelmed, as he had feared, and sat with him as he read his father's statement to her. Michael's relationship with the suitcase and its contents was intensifying, and I felt that he would benefit from an in-person session.

He arrived smiling, with his suitcase, saying he felt relief and a sense of freedom in taking it out of his home. He had feared an accident occurring on-route, which might damage the suitcase and its precious contents, but he also told me that the 20-minute journey had been less fraught and complicated by anxiety than it would have been in the past. I took this as an indication of significant healing.

Feeling awe for the presence of the suitcase and the significance of the session, I suggested we proceed slowly to explore his relationship with the suitcase, which we did through discussion and contact with the past and present. Towards the end of the session, Michael, with a smile, opened the suitcase and produced an image of his parents on their wedding day in England. I was struck by Henryk's resolute expression, standing with Maria for their new life in the UK.

As the session approached its end, we talked a little about the connections between our histories, the family pictures in my room and those in his suitcase. Michael asked me to send him the Introduction and Chapter 1 of this book. The following session would also be in person.

Michael arrived without the suitcase. Laughing, he explained this was because of the stormy weather and a fear that a tree could fall on his car and damage the suitcase and its contents. He judged this worry as 'absurd', but I voiced my appreciation of the preciousness of the suitcase and its documents.

Referring to his reading in Chapter 1 of my synchronistic experiences in Salonika, Michael told me of Jessica seeing a similar suitcase to his of 1950s vintage on a wall near his home and worrying it might be Michael's. It was not, but rather a remarkable coincidence, which we took as an affirmation of the significance of the work and the connection between himself and Jessica through this process. In the past week, they had decided to read through the suitcase's contents again.

Michael had recently found a citation concerning his father in the academic document about Stutthof Concentration Camp and the evacuations from it in the maritime 'death marches' (*Stutthof Maritime Evacuations Project,* International Holocaust Remembrance Alliance, 2021). With this discovery, I sensed the healing potency of Michael's learning that his father's traumas had been signified, recorded and held. Michael was developing a different relationship with the family past. Instead of being overwhelmed by existential despair and aloneness-pain, he was exploring and processing it within relationship, and his enriched present life.

He reflected with me weighty feelings of excitement, duty and stress concerning the option of sharing, with an archive, the manuscript his father had left for him. In an earlier session, using DBR with the activating stimulus of the grip of his parents' histories, he connected with the perspective that his father didn't want him to be crushed by their past. Michael wondered more freely: As his father had formally signed the manuscript, perhaps he wished it to be seen in the public domain?

I reflected back to Michael the vitality I saw in him and contrasted it with his statement when we first met, of the therapy being about the 'endgame' of his life. He stressed that my transgenerational approach had been the key to his healing. I felt moved, sensing our work within the transpersonal field of soul, to be larger than both of us and an honouring of our ancestors whilst being present in the moment to reflect together and freer in Janet's term, to 'triumph' over phantoms of tragedies past. I was taken aback as he thanked me for 'letting me [him] in the room' *vis a vis* my Jewish/holocaust background, indicating an attitude that seemed to diminish the significance of the immense suffering, fortitude and heroism of his dear parents, and the burden it had been his fate to carry. Concerning this attitude of discount, Michael has subsequently explored the formative impact upon him of his uncle's celebration as a war hero of the RAF, overshadowing his father's travails and accomplishments.

Due to my having COVID, the following session was online. Michael told me his relationship with the suitcase was changing, now seeing its rich historical contents as a resource, a 'toolbox', in his unfolding journey of processing, disentanglement and personal integration. He reflected on how he had seriously considered destroying the box and its contents earlier in our work together. In the past week, he had spent many hours studying the academic piece concerning Stutthof Concentration Camp and the maritime death marches (*Stutthof Maritime Evacuations Project*, International Holocaust Remembrance Alliance, 2021) and had placed it in the box with all the family documents and photographs.

Honouring His Parents: The Healing of Self and History

From earlier in our work together, Michael resumed exploration concerning being witness to his parents' ugly conflicts with each other, such as his mother's allegations of infidelity against his father and the latter's response of intense distress. Despite his anguish in needing to speak of these experiences, he completed his voicing of them as a movement of release from enmeshment with his parents. In this cycle of experience and personal expression, I was impacted by Michael's care for both his parents, in liberated, enlightened love of them as their son.

Michael continued to study his father's statement, and I was deeply moved by his sharing a description of Henryk's moment of liberation by allied soldiers. He expressed sadness for his father's reserved attitude and the lack of acknowledgement concerning his role in the Polish resistance, survival of Stutthof Concentration Camp and the 'death marches at sea' and creation (with Michael's mother) of a new life in the UK. Michael conveyed with feeling how his father was overshadowed, by the celebrated status of his uncle as a pilot in the RAF. By expressing his father's deserving of the honours accorded to his uncle, Michael was undoing a personal and familial fixed gestalt of self-suppression, a retroflection of energy and so also connecting with his own value for a healing of self and history (you may wish to refer back to my exploration of Gestalt therapy, in Chapter 4). To repeat the words of Beaumont quoted in Chapter 6: 'When we are able to remember our father's essence we do better… and our father does better' (2012, p. 33).

In alignment with his process of individuation, Michael told me that he was no longer going to be governed by 'shoulds' and specifically related this to advice provided by friends with respect to the possible release of the document to an archive or institution. He would take time to consider the various options for placing his father's statement into the public domain. Michael also appreciated my suggestion that he hold firmly to his appreciation of his father's value with organisations he might approach, to consider if their attitude and conduct expressed the depth of respect due to him and his statement.

In summary, to repeat Hillman's words I quoted in Chapter 6: in this way, Michael is honouring the presence of the dead, 'hearing [of] the voices of history' (2013, p. 151), and perhaps enabling healing for them as he grows through self-actualising engagement with the world.

Michael's increasing freedom and strength of self are reflected in several ways. He has a renewed vitality for life, in great contrast to his position at the beginning of therapy, when he was strongly attracted to suicide. He has resumed his activity within the arts, regularly attending meetings to pursue his interests. In his developing relationship with Jessica, he can listen to and appreciate her feelings and needs while being faithful and expressive of his own. This is a significant indication of his healing and disentanglement from the fate of his mother: in being self-present within a relationship rather than being overwhelmed by feelings of guilt for another's discomfort and/or withdrawal.

Michael recently told me, 'I think maybe I've got to the top of the mountain and am on the descent', meaning he has faced issues which, at the start of therapy, he didn't think he would or could. The 'descent' is the process of integration, honouring his parents, the past and living in the present time. Our work continues.

Note

1 Poland, as a country, ceased to exist in the late eighteenth century and was partitioned between three Empires until the end of the First World War: the German Empire, the Russian Empire and the Austro-Hungarian Empire. Poland was re-established as a country in 1918. Before the start of the Second World War, Nazi Germany and the Soviet Union made a secret Pact to abolish Poland as a country again and partition it between them. At the beginning of the War, in September 1939, the Germans invaded from the West and the Russians from the East. Following the Second World War, Poland's existence as a country was confirmed, but within very different borders from its shape between 1918 and 1939.

References

Bako, T. & Zana, K. (2020) *Transgenerational Trauma and Therapy: The Transgenerational Atmosphere*. Abingdon, Oxon: Routledge.

Beaumont, H. (2012) *Toward a Spiritual Psychotherapy: Soul as a Dimension of Experience*. Berkeley, CA: North Atlantic Books.

Hillman, J. & Shamdasani, S. (2013) *Lament of the Dead: Psychology after Jung's Red Book*. New York: Norton.

Straede, T., Overby, M.J. & Möller, R. (2021) *Academic Report: Stutthof Maritime Evacuations Project*. International Holocaust Remembrance Alliance: A project conducted 2020–21 by the University of Southern Denmark (Odense), the Neuengamme Concentration Camp Memorial (Hamburg), The Viking Ship Museum (Roskilde) and JD Contractors (Holstebro) in cooperation with the Muzeum Stutthof (Sztutowo).

Chapter 8

Trauma, Identity Politics and Psychotherapy

My perspective on this contemporary theme is intimately related to my soul
connection with my ancestors, their dehumanisation and murder, and my drive
to express and aid redemptive affirmation of human be-ing in their honour.
I offer this chapter, as I do the whole book, with the wish that it may be of use.
My intention in sharing personal experience is to include myself
and my own potential for destructive reactivity, irrationality, and self-
righteousness endemic in the human condition with respect to personal and
group identity. In doing so, I am seeking to avoid implicitly placing myself
above and separate from others and thereby mirroring and contributing to
the process of splitting and division.
I believe the more that we can appreciate our frailties, flaws, and
connectedness, the better the prospects for humanity in resolving division,
conflict, and violence and reducing unnecessary suffering.

In this chapter, I offer reflections concerning the interface between three elements intrinsic to the therapeutic encounter:

- Trauma.
- The ways we experience and treat each other.
- Therapeutic release from such suffering, which can enable connection and reconnection to ourselves and other people.

I believe unresolved trauma impedes mutual understanding and contact, which, as a consequence, reinforces the negative beliefs and perceptions that we carry.

I am aware of my capacity in the context of the enduring effects of trauma to subtly dissociate and feel self-righteous hostility towards the Other. I remember feeling intense pain and outrage when I reflected on the transgenerational trauma and personal memories of antisemitism that I have experienced. During these times, I found myself identifying with the suffering of my ancestors, but I also noticed within myself the emergence of a hateful and objectifying attitude towards other people. And, at times, the collision of this experience with assertions that I am a beneficiary of white privilege affected and amplified my sense of vulnerability

DOI: 10.4324/9781003456438-9

and persecution. I believe the term used within identity politics of 'white fragility' (Di-Angelo, 2018), which might be applied to such a disclosure, occludes understanding of complex human processes, including those of trauma. Through therapy, I was able to heal from the depth of my trauma and enjoy an easing of such effects.

Holding an open and compassionate attitude towards each person, irrespective of their appearance and background, is a prerequisite for healing dialogue and work. From personal reflection and my work with clients, what I have found to be of great importance is a commitment towards holding as primary and fundamental both our individual uniqueness and collective oneness as sentient beings. As a proponent of transpersonal psychotherapy, Rowan used the TARDIS from the British science fiction TV series 'Doctor Who' as a metaphor for us humans to proclaim on his website:

> ...the person is a bit like the TARDIS – pretty unimpressive on the outside, but practically infinite on the inside, with huge resources and immense untrodden ways. The person is not a poor limited worm on the face of the earth, but a being of great potential and magical connections.

Trauma, Identity and Object Relations

I appreciate the immense depth of trauma carried by people of colour, from colonisation and slavery and their contemporary re-enactments, and the persisting forms of oppression, persecution and injustice which, having white skin, I have not had visited upon me. Indeed, whilst it compounded my experience of toxic shame and a further shrinking of self, I avoided beatings at school by hiding my Jewishness, something people of colour cannot do. For example, on a school coach, a group of hostile and aggressive boys turned to my classmates and asked: 'Is he a Yid?' They answered, 'No, he's all right', and I stayed silent, feeling frightened and humiliated but remaining physically unharmed.

I recognise that our society is riven with deep and wide-ranging inequities and inequalities and that it is crucial that they are identified, named and challenged, and that we consider race, religion, gender, sexuality and other forms of socialised identity as significant and important to explore. However, giving priority to these categories of identity[1] can cause us to overlook our ultimate spiritual unity to bring or exacerbate division and contribute to conflict and oppression. With this attitude, there can occur a perpetuation (sometimes *via* inversion) of an object relation of the oppressor-oppressed or perpetrator-victim. It is evident in the unjust, oppressive and murderous conduct of governments worldwide towards marginalised groups and also in the manner with which we perceive and interact with one another.

The concept of object relations was developed within psychoanalytic psychotherapy to understand child development, psychodynamics and relational processes (Hughes, 1989). I am using it to describe where a fixed binary template of our relationship with and between ourselves and others is active, limiting our capacity for contact, empathy and compassion.

This sort of alternating object relation (called by Racker, 1982, p. 140, 'paranoid ping pong') can be inferred in the ongoing tragedy of the Middle East (Personal communication: Sills, 2024). It is also present within the field of psychotherapy through the application of intersectional theory, which I will discuss later in this chapter with respect to the work of Dwight Turner. The following quote from Robin Di-Angelo is an example of the inversion and perpetuation of a persecutory object relation in response to the oppression and persecution of people of colour:

> I believe that *white progressives cause the most daily damage to people of color.* I define a white progressive as anyone who thinks he or she is not racist, or is less racist, or is in the "choir," or already "gets it".
>
> (2018, p. 5)

The grouping and attribution of blame to people in this way (amplified by the apparently ironic placement of the label 'progressive' within the discussion of racism – a categorically *regressive* process) reveal a perspective characteristic of splitting and projection. Substituting 'white progressive' with another label, such as 'immigrant' or 'blue-collar', reveals the underlining, dehumanising and corrosive effect of this accusation against people, each of whom has the right to be met with respect rather than derision.

In the following passage, Beaumont reflects upon attitudes consequent of trauma that perpetuate conflict and suffering and the risk posed by movements towards confluence with collective trauma implicit in Di-Angelo's attitude:

> A documentary film was made in Slovenia shortly after the political entity of Yugoslavia dissolved. A cave had been discovered in which 17, 000 corpses were buried in three layers. The first layer contained dead nationalists who had been killed by the communists. The second layer contained communists who had been murdered with the help of the Gestapo. The top layer were nationalists who had been killed after the war by the communists who had returned to power. A young man whose murdered relatives were found in the middle layer was interviewed in the film. He was asked if the acts of revenge would ever come to an end. His answer was dramatic: –
>
> "As long as we can still hear the weeping of our mothers for their dead sons, and see their tears, there can be no peace."
>
> When we listen to this young man, we can see the result of unfinished grief and the corresponding limitations placed on soul. We have to ask which mothers he is looking at, and which dead? This young man was certainly suffering, but his inability to allow grief to do its work threatens to perpetuate suffering.
>
> (Beaumont, 2012, p. 167)

Unity, Alienation and Transgenerational Trauma

Psychotherapy needs to be a process of contact and engagement with the whole of a person's experience, including those of the transpersonal and transgenerational dimensions. Embracing difference means holding our ultimate unity as souls and soul. One's social, racial, tribal, sexual and gender identity are aspects of this totality, and each can be significant in a person's therapeutic journey. However, when a person's appearance and social identity are the primary determinants of their own and others' beliefs about them and how they should be addressed, an objectifying and alienating process is in train, enacting an oppression and repression of the soul, perhaps paralleling patterns embedded from innumerable generations and reflecting the shadow aspect of the human condition. This is counter to the spirit and endeavour of psychotherapy, for it is a movement away from engagement with the depth of our being, relationally, intrapsychically and spiritually, to accommodate an established or counter-cultural hegemony which has the conceit to impose a definition of who we are upon us.

I believe such alienated social and political processes flow from historic and collective trauma, challenging our ability to be present and open to meet ourselves and others. That which we carry from past and contemporary experiences of our family, race, gender and culture can be overwhelming. Thomas Hubl, in his book *Healing Collective Trauma* (2020), describes how our perception of the world can be distorted because of an 'unresolved past' (p. 9) and psychic fragmentation caused by trauma, which warps our experience of space-time. Because of our nature and form and the reality of human history, we are all affected to some extent by collective traumas of the past. Thus, we are vulnerable to mistaking the present for the past and can have difficulty distinguishing between current experiences and those of the past, which are still active within our psyche and soma. In this context, separating trauma from its psychological, historical and spiritual aspects to exclusively attend to it as a political issue will result in it being neglected. It's important to practise psychotherapy with understanding and differentiation between ongoing experiences of oppression, injustice and persecution and those of the past; and the current circumstances and changing challenges which a client faces, including new opportunities for connection, contact and relationship.

As cited in Chapter 4, in *Transgenerational Trauma and Therapy: The Transgenerational Atmosphere* (2020), Bako and Zana offer an analysis of the intrapsychic, relational and systemic dynamics within traumatised families from which offspring carry transgenerational trauma – the unresolved past and warped experience of space-time named by Hubl (2020). This occurs *via* a familial 'transgenerational atmosphere' and 'we-experience' redolent of past horrors (Bako & Zana, 2020). It is a self-perpetuating domain of trauma, from which there is insufficient contact and connection with and trust in the current environment. This book is based on work with Holocaust survivors and succeeding generations. I believe it provides a vehicle for the understanding and addressing of the issues and challenges facing all groups who have been subjected to oppression and persecution.

I am concerned about the potential of we who live with transgenerational trauma to carry dogma and ideology which splits the world into friend or foe, good or bad, to occlude self-awareness, contact with others and access to healing. Such splitting is a self-protective response to the experience and perception of threat, fear and the unknown. Melanie Klein, with the concept of the 'Paranoid schizoid position' (1946), identified this primitive propensity within the human condition, through which we react to discomfort by splitting, projecting and discharging unwanted feelings (the 'bad object') onto the environment and other people. She contrasts this with the more mature process of the 'Depressive position', through which there is acceptance, containment and self-regulation of discomfort in our experiences and behaviour towards the environment and others.

Intersectional Theory and Trauma Therapy

To reiterate, politics which focus on identity can be catalysts for personal and collective regression to the paranoid-schizoid position and a deflection from necessary healing and contact, as observed by Beaumont in the passage I quoted earlier. I appreciate the identity politics of the 'left' as a discourse concerned with oppression, persecution, deprivation and injustice suffered by people *via* 'intersections' (Turner, 2021) in their social, economic and political circumstances. This perspective can facilitate insights and the expansion of our awareness as part of the process of psychotherapy, but it is not a substitute for engagement with our internal worlds and the process necessary for the healing of trauma. In previous chapters, I have explored the enduring effects of trauma and our inner experience of them. I am concerned that in the absence of a holistic approach, the lens of intersectionality may support their perpetuation by politicising rather than aiding healing and resolving of archaic oppressed-oppressor and victim-perpetrator object relations towards the Other, which we carry from past traumas. Beaumont, here, reflects, with applicability to systemic and transgenerational traumas of oppression and persecution, on the perpetrator-victim object relation within family systems and our need to release ourselves from them, in order to become free of resonances of victimhood carried from our histories:

> Together they form a system and are one systemic whole…As long as we identify ourselves as victims we have to hold on to our perpetrators. If we want to stop feeling like a victim, we have to let go of our perpetrators…This means that we are faced with the task of changing our sense of identity, our sense of who we are.
>
> (2012, pp. 20–21)

Intersections of Privilege and Otherness in Counselling and Psychotherapy: Mockingbird (2021) by Dwight Turner is an important book. Through the sharing of his own experiences, it is deeply impactful and moving, with respect to the truly unimaginable suffering of people of colour over many centuries up to the present day. I understand it to be immersed in and concerned with that aspect of our human condition from which we, individually and collectively, create and repeat oppression, suffering and trauma (with its enduring effects) by 'othering' and the interpersonal and systemic abuse of power and privilege towards particular groups of people, such as people of colour, Jews, women, disabled people and those of the LGBTQ+ community. However, when Turner's intersectional-psychodynamic approach is applied to trauma, it can overlook the complexity and depth of the phenomenon and our potential for healing and realisation of our ultimate spiritual unity: as I, We and Thou. In this way, I consider Turner's view that '…the intersectional nature of difference is core to our identity as human beings' (p. 12) is one which is limiting and maintains rather than eases those object relations of oppressed-oppressor and victim-persecutor which no longer match our circumstances. There are serious implications and issues that flow from Turner's intersectional analysis of psychological processes:

- In his theory, the casework he presents and the sharing of his own journey, Turner appears to posit that our psychological processes are reducible to the intersectional dynamics of power, privilege and otherness: 'the intersectional nature of identity' (p. 106). My earnest plea is that we refrain from defining ourselves and others in this way. This is because respecting and holding the profound depth and immanence within and between us is vital for the healing of trauma, for personal unfolding, and, more broadly, for loving attention towards the catastrophic violent conflicts which encircle our world.
- Turner's philosophy contrasts with a humanist perspective in its prioritising of difference over our core identity as human beings, for dissonance to be more important than our commonality as individual manifestations from the 'ground of being' (as held by both religious and secular humanism), of which we each are an expression and part. This perspective restricts the potential for open exploration and spiritual depth in the practice of psychotherapy.

Turner offers the following vignette concerning transgenerational trauma from his research, which I believe he misinterprets through his intersectional formulation of psychodynamic processes with respect to self and others and the inner 'death drive against the other' (Turner, p. 86). Alejandra, a Jewish-Venezuelan participant in Turner's research, recalls and visualises an episode of antisemitism perpetrated upon her by a taxi driver. This led her to feel a sensation in her throat and to then connect with an experience of watching the film 'The Pianist' (which is concerned with the Warsaw Ghetto and the Holocaust), in which SS officers throw a Jewish grandfather in a wheelchair out of a window:

> A totally defenceless person…I'm just, it makes me tearful as I couldn't watch the film after that (inaudible)…I couldn't stand it.
>
> (p. 87)

Alejandra has uncovered the memory of watching this terrible film scene from the recollection, visualising and somatic sensing of the antisemitic 'microaggression' from the taxi driver concerning the bombing of a Jewish centre in Buenos Aires and the deaths it caused. This tragedy had occurred whilst she was in the city. The encounter with the taxi driver is a common example of the experiences of Jews with regard to antisemitism, transgenerational trauma and intertwined patterns of survival. This is exemplified in Alejandra's statement: 'I just made a comment then I shut up. And then I felt bad about it' (p. 86), which is an expression that conveys thousands of years of suffering expulsions, persecution and pogroms culminating in the Holocaust, to which her consciousness had turned. However, Turner interprets Alejandra's connecting of her experience and 'ambivalence' with the taxi driver to that of her viewing the murder of the Jewish grandfather by the SS in 'The Pianist' in the following way:

> Her ambivalence is also apparent... in the struggle to both watch and avoid the harrowing scenes held in the film, her rejection of the chance to sit with her partner and watch the film matching her inability to speak up...It is as if in not speaking up for her culture in the taxi she has unconsciously internalised the 'murder' of her Jewish sense of self.
>
> (p. 88)

Turner then asserts:

> Her tears during our meeting also resonated with the pain of this story, the pain of this act of psychological self-harm. What is less apparent is the internalised abuser within this scene, the aspect that does the murdering, that strives for something more privileged...it is not that Alejandra is an abusive person...this internalised abuser already resides within her, like a sub-personality.
>
> (p. 88)

And a few sentences later, he states:

> This alternative perspective on her unconscious, internalised sense of superiority and its destruction of that which makes her culturally different, could also be seen to be driven by the same envy discussed previously; a deeply internalised envy [from the taxi-driver] that is driven to self-destroy.
>
> (p. 89)

In these passages, I believe Turner fails to demonstrate an understanding of Alejandra's distress and the depth and profundity of collective transgenerational trauma, which I have explored in previous chapters. For example, he treats her upset and sadness with the following words: 'her rejection of the chance to sit with her partner and watch the film' (p. 88). Also, he applies a forensic attitude towards Alejandra in his use of the term 'internalised abuser'. I suggest that Alejandra's response to the film wasn't, as Turner argues, an attempt to maintain her connection and identification with privilege but an authentic experience of distress, flight and dissociation in response to material, that touched her 'internalised transgenerational wounds' (Turner, p. 89). I think the first few words of the following sentence convey a feeling of insecurity from Turner concerning the interpretation he is offering the reader with respect to Alejandra's connecting of the two scenes:

Yet, whilst this might all seem strange, what I am highlighting here is the factor where the aggressiveness, in fact that and the hatred, of the taxi-driver has become implanted within Alejandra to such an extent that this event...which occurred many years ago still brought up such a vivid image of self-hatred and self-destruction.

(p. 89)

I suggest Turner's sense that his analysis could 'seem strange' is because *he* has 'implanted' a notion into the discussion. This is through his concentration on the single interaction with the taxi driver and its effects, which minimises the reality and depth of Alejandra's Jewish transgenerational trauma that was activated by and which connected the two scenes.

In addition to applying my knowledge and experience of working with trauma, I remember my own viewing of the film and finding that scene unbearably painful and wishing to move away and flee. At that moment, I saw the grandfather as one of my murdered ancestors. There was activation of the transgenerational trauma within my body and soul and connection to the transpersonal collective unconscious, interactive field (which I discussed in Chapter 4) concerning the impossible, appalling dilemmas Jews faced during the Holocaust and their responses to dissociate (*e.g.* to find a way to disbelieve the horrific reports they were hearing), freeze, flee, hide or fight.

It is inappropriate for us to pass judgement upon the experience of the millions of people who faced that horror, and the precious few who survived, nor the succeeding generations by whom it is carried with the fixed gestalts that were forged in that abyss of annihilation, to be shared, with psychotherapists in therapy rooms. I believe the therapeutic relationship is a field of collaboration between therapist and client, a space for opening to the depth of such trauma, which had not yet been previously expressible or expressed. This needs to be in place for psychotherapy with all complex, transgenerational and collective traumas.

I readily acknowledge my subjectivity in the interpretation I am offering with respect to Alejandra and her psychological process. I suggest Turner also also drew upon his own profound suffering in the construction of the intersectional interpretation he is offering. Irrespective of our opinions, Alejandra needed what Carl Rogers called 'unconditional positive regard' (1967), empathy and compassion, which seems to have been muted beneath Turner's theory. Furthermore, it is important to distinguish between the practice of therapy and acts of unmasking (Baehr, 2019)[2] as evoked by Turner's words to which I again refer: 'this internalised abuser resides within her, like a sub-personality', which is held by a tautology through his repeated assertion of intersectional theory.

Both our philosophies of therapy have been formed *a priori* from key assumptions, mine concerning the essence and the ultimate unity of soul: one of Turner's is a philosophically materialist belief in the primacy of the interpersonal and political environment with respect to identity and self. However, in my view, instead of aiding insight, such a materialist, intersectional and conflict-based perspective concerning trauma can be a buttress for avoiding therapeutic challenges. To heal from trauma, we must face the reality of our condition, as the person in Beaumont's vignette needed to do, for the relief of suffering and the cessation of a cycle of violence. I have reflected upon the legacy of experiences of antisemitism in my childhood and how, in later years, the memory of those frightening and humiliating experiences, combined with my transgenerational trauma, putrefied within me to become a hateful, objectifying grudge towards people who happened to be gentile. In the process of healing from my traumas, I needed to face and awaken from this pathological and negative attitude towards the other. Antisemitism is as virulent as ever in this world, and it is present in my life; however, phantoms of traumas past no longer so powerfully pollute my worldview and attitudes towards other people.

Trauma and Group Identifications

Psychological and spiritual trauma is a consequence of experiences in which a person has been overwhelmed beyond their functional capacity to stay present and available within the unfolding now. A process of dissociation, intrapsychic splitting and projecting of disturbance have occurred and are in place as our organism and soul respond, seeking to regain or retain a sense of safety and control. There may also be a drive to relieve feelings of shame and deficiency through the projection onto others of the sense of 'basic fault' (Balint, 1979), with an amelioration sought through withdrawal and or aggressive, hate-infused thinking and action. We will strive to cope with the wounding and contamination of the soul, but our fundamental trust in self, others and the world has been fractured.

Traumatic material and experiences, including those from the transgenerational and transpersonal domains, may carry profound insights and understanding.

It is essential that psychotherapy facilitates, supports and affirms people's abilities, needs and rights to challenge oppression. However, these need to be appreciated in balance with the person's circumstances and careful attention to archaic intrapsychic dynamics, beliefs and survival strategies formed in response to past traumas. Through the latter, we are prone to miss deeper contact with ourselves and the opportunities for healing, nourishing and reparative contact with people we meet.

It is important to understand both the inner and sociological dynamics which distort and distract us from opportunities for healing contact and the movement of our souls towards contact and healing:

> ...people fall into patterns of discord, struggling for power, triggering one another, operating with victim/oppressor dynamics, and ultimately feeling the pain of separation. Yet, repetition of these unconscious patterns is the steady call of the soul to feel into, acknowledge, embrace and heal.
>
> (Hubl, 2020, p. 155)

When the person is ready for engagement with the current environment with an open attitude of connection and relationship, the healing of past traumas can commence along with a dissolving of and moving beyond a perpetrator-victim object relation. This is why my meetings with Volker at Auschwitz-Birkenau and via Skype, which I described in Chapter 1, were so significant to me.

The experience of collective contact and support is very significant for people living with trauma and oppression. Still, the need for such holding and understanding can guide a person towards people and groups with a familiar, phobic social consciousness – a 'we-experience' as described by Zana and Bako (2020). Such contact can reinforce and affirm cognitions and defensive behaviours rooted in trauma, with a collective language and merging against perceived demon others. In this way, in-group identification and communication can become an alienating vehicle of defence against the 'bad object' (Klein, 1946) projected onto the other, to reinforce a trauma-based apprehension of opportunities for broader social and personal meeting – which hold the potential to be healing mismatch experiences, against the haunting past and allow an expansion of relational-consciousness in the present moment.

The Damaging Potential of Concepts

In the realm of trauma, words are compelling, and I am concerned about their damaging potential. I wrote in Chapter 1 how this matter impacted my childhood home, with the British National Health Service's destructive application of concepts and allied treatments, which exacerbated the suffering in my family. Thus, I am vigilant with respect to the potential of concepts to objectify and lead to harm rather than support understanding and awareness. White privilege is an important concept, and obsessive-compulsive disorder, attention deficit hyperactivity disorder and narcissism are valid clinical terms. However, when they are misused as means of verbal attack, they are damaging in their deriding and discounting of a person's experience and self.

The term white privilege can support a liberating opening to and mobilisation of awareness concerning the profound and transgenerational dimensions of experience with respect to anti-black racism, the breadth and depth of horrific suffering it caused and causes, and the benefits accrued by those seen as white. It is a term with both deep historical and contemporary relevance, and when used with clarity and focus, it uncovers and describes important truths. However, if it is elongated (Baehr, 2019, 2021) beyond its usefulness in personal relationships and the discourse of identity politics, as in the lines I quoted earlier from Di-Angelo, it will perpetuate the objectification of human beings, conflict and the traumas people suffer as a result.

A person's experience of direct or introjected pressure to organise reflections about their life and personal experience in alignment with a concept is a form of oppression. This may occur from the experience of cumulative judgement and disrespect, such as in the contexts of bullying on social media and domestic coercive control. They will likely have been a recipient and vehicle of the bad object, projected onto them by another person or people. In effect, the person has been subjected to:

> Attentional violence …[which] is to not see another person, another human being, in terms of who they really are, or for their highest future possibility. When who you truly are goes unseen by society, a form of violence is inflicted upon you.
>
> (Scharmer in Hubl, 2020, p. 176)

In the vignette I offer below from my work with Carrie, the process is as important as the content, it being one of objectification and bullying; oppressive behaviour which misuses concepts and categories of identity:

Carrie told me that a colleague at work spoke dismissively and disrespectfully towards her and her female colleagues. The colleague sought to buttress his aggressive, domineering behaviour with reference to his experience and identity, articulating objectifying assumptions about Carrie (and her colleagues) from his perception of their gender and social identities. For Carrie, the process with this colleague had a toxic resonance with experiences from several aspects of her life (as we will see in Chapter 9), in which she had been subjected to oppressive behaviour and the discounting of her human value and experience. I sought to be alongside Carrie in her sharing of this situation with me as she explored her experience of the colleague's 'attentional violence' and its meaning to her in relation to her personal journey.

Such attentional violence can be especially harmful and destructive to a person who carries the wounds of humiliation and shaming in their soul. It can cause a relapse into disconnection from self and their personal value and the fracturing of a precious, fragile self-confidence and inner trust, perhaps nurtured over many years. I have worked with clients who discounted and deflected from exploration of their personal experience, because of having been subjected to and introjecting as accurate, the use of words abusive of them.

People who use words dissonantly, without human connection and awareness of another, are likely suffering and living with a disconnection from the self. Bollas in *Meaning and Melancholia: Life in the Age of Bewilderment* (2018) offers an analysis of alienated thinking and use of words as a result of: 'cumulative oppression',

> When people who have been physically tortured are freed from their captors, the way they walk and try to speak shows that their way of being has been compromised. Those who are otherwise oppressed over long periods of time may also show changes in the way they think, talk and relate.…
>
> (2018, p. 67)

In psychotherapy, the healing route concerning the aggressive expression of such suffering is *via* the forming and work of a therapeutic alliance of compassionate exploration.

Positive and Negative Paranoia

Bollas provides understanding of processes behind the attritional use of words, from a borderline split consequent of the fragmenting effects of Western history: the slaughter and 'moral catastrophes of colonialism' (p. 18), two world wars and its manifestation in contemporary far-right and far-left ideologies.

He describes this split in Western society and consciousness as being evident since the First World War. 'A decade after this, psychiatry would propose a new formation: a self divided down the middle, one part that idealized the world and another that hated it' (p. 29), and from both world wars came '...a waning of self-reflection, self-examination and self-accountability...we abandoned our conscience and entered an underworld populated by the most destructive elements of human nature' (p. 121).

Bollas identifies the orientation of 'positive paranoia' within the ideological right-wing, this being an active, hateful and persecutory attitude towards other groups of people. And on the 'left', and within the practice of identity politics, he identifies its counterpart:

> ...negative paranoia...where selves become ostensibly empty of personal views. These are replaced with a mission: to embody a blameless self, opposed to the vulgarities of life and allied with all that is virtuous...[to]... occupy a position of sublime innocence, using common phrases to denounce others, implicitly exalting the self.
>
> (2018, pp. 106–7)

This self-righteousness mirrors that of the positive paranoia on the 'right' supported by a discourse that obscures its conceit. To this orientation, Bollas attributes behaviours such as the passive-aggressive use of 'dead face' and a vigilant, combative response to perceived 'micro-aggressions' emanating from the identified hostile other.[3]

Right-wing positive paranoia and left-wing negative paranoia are manifestations of a fractured world in which the humane flow of proportionate, personal exchange and dialogue is missing within a vicious circle of suffering and conflict. In this process of attrition, the issues needing to be addressed are obscured; their significance and function being disowned *via* projection onto the other, possibly with violence, causing the forms of traumas which I am addressing in this book.

Bollas reflects: 'To talk to one's presumed enemies is also to engage in a conversation with oneself; to find the good that is resident in all people is perhaps the most difficult task of all. But we owe it to ourselves' (2018, p. xxx); for a 'new form of collective understanding in which humans can turn once more again towards becoming humane beings' (2018, p. 129). The function of the psychotherapy I have described in this book aligns with this view, with respect to the need to engage compassionately with the client in the healing of trauma, providing relief from suffering which is not derived from the discharging of the bad object on the demonised other but, instead, a return to the experience of wholeness and sense of commonality with other sentient beings. In the next section, I share a vignette from my work with a client, which illustrates such a healing process.

Sabine

Sabine is a German woman who was born in the 1970s, a student of the Diamond Approach with the Ridhwan School, and a senior, highly successful medical professional. Sabine had experienced difficulty in maintaining relationships, both personal and professional. She has carried a heightened sense of vulnerability and vigilance against dismissal and rejection by others. Her experience of conflict and disagreement with other people had activated excruciating feelings of inner wounding and toxic shame. In our work together, we had a warm and strong therapeutic alliance, which included a sharing of our experiences of each other that supported Sabine's exploration of herself and her relationships.

Sabine began the session with a check-in, mentioning that her relationships with both her partner and a colleague, 'A', had improved. With her partner, she had become more able to recognise and appreciate his qualities of stability and acceptance, with these no longer blending in her mind with the traumatic, formative childhood experiences of her family. She saw that her beliefs and reactive patterns were central to the issues in their relationship. Sabine told me that with colleague A, there had been a coming together and softening in their relationship, following intense distrust and friction over more than two years. A piece of family constellation work with an ongoing group, of which she was a member, had been helpful. In it, she saw a connection with issues she carried from her relationship with her father, of rejection, dismissal and judgement, and, with her siblings, of competition.

Sabine then moved the conversation to speak of conflict with another colleague, B, by whom she continued to feel rejected. I suggested that rather than an attitude of rejection, fear might be the factor that influenced colleague B to push back a meeting Sabine had proposed for them. I shared my sense of her power and the experience of sometimes feeling jolted back during our dialogues. Sabine recognised this and the possibility of a vicious circle of mutual reactivity between colleague B and herself, causing them to feel alienated from each other and leaving her feeling hurt and rejected.

She began to speak about a part of herself she calls the 'Soldier', who is efficient and strong, and 'gets things done'. 'I like him', she said. I reflected back my feeling for her German family, and the tumult of the first half of the twentieth century which they had endured. Sabine then told me of an incident sometime after the end of the Second World War: occupying, allied soldiers visited the family farm and told her father they were going to take his only horse. The horse was essential for the functioning of the farm. He confronted the soldiers, telling them that in order to take the horse 'You will have to kill me', and they relented from their demand.

I suggested to Sabine that she tell her soldier the current date. She then looked shocked, because she found that whilst he kind of knew the war was over, he felt the time period he was inhabiting was 1940 to 1945. She continued to reflect upon her liking of him; he got things done, but, he also frightened people. I expressed my respect for him, again sharing my feelings of resonance and appreciation of her family's drive to survive through the desperate course of the early and middle parts of the twentieth century. She looked moved and said, 'this is special' [because of…] 'your background' (mine, as a Jew), and she thought of her Israeli friend and their visit to Yad Vashem. I told her of my German friend, Dorle, our retreats at Auschwitz and our monthly Skype meetings. This was a poignant I-Thou moment, in which we were both deeply affected.

Sabine then said the soldier had put his gun down. She reflected with sadness about feeling 'one is doing the right thing, but…': I again reflected back a sense of being caught in tumultuous, overwhelming processes. As Sabine relaxed, we talked some more, and she asked her soldier if he would take advice from other parts of her before acting. He thought this would be good but was also a little wary and cynical. I suggested patience and gentleness with his learning about and coming to terms with this different time. *I suggested Sabine tell her soldier that she is doing well in her life*, in order to reassure him about decision-making through a collaboration with other parts of herself.

Sabine, in contrast to most previous sessions in which I needed to provide holding and containment for the ending, said she felt the work was 'complete' for the day, and her body felt heavy but grounded. She smiled in response to my request to write about our work together for this book, twice saying, 'That would please me'.

Following her reading of the above vignette, Sabine shared this important, significant information and reflection:

> The soldier also said he is tired of fighting and does not want to fight anymore. He felt betrayed for fighting for the wrong thing / reason (which I think you considered by writing "one is doing the right thing, but…"). The soldier felt that he was wronged by trying to do the right thing… and this is also how I felt / feel a lot of the time (work as well as outside of work). The soldier knew the war was over but did not know how to live in this world.

This final line from Sabine poignantly expresses much that I have sought to convey in this chapter and book concerning the issues and gifts we carry as a species concerning our ability to live and be fully present in this world as beings (to repeat Rowan's words) 'of great potential and magical connections'.

Notes

1 Peter Baehr, in 'Are "They" Us? The Intellectuals' Role in Creating Division' (2021) succinctly describes the practice of elongation, whereby a concept is extended and applied beyond its potential to bring beneficent understanding to an issue.

2 In 'The Unmasking Style in Social Theory' (2019), Baehr explains and critiques unmasking.

3 It is important to distinguish the interlocking, intrapsychically and relationally alienated processes described by Bollas and summarised by me, from situations and contexts in which it is imperative for a person or group to respond effectively to attack and violating behaviours, including micro-aggressions. I know the latter to be a significant feature in many abusive, corrosive and traumatising scenarios.

References

Baehr, P. (2021) Are "they" us? The intellectuals' role in creating division. *HA: Journal of the Hannah Arendt Center* 2021, Vol. 8, pp. 66–72.

Baehr, P. (2019) *The Unmasking Style in Social Theory: (Classical and Contemporary Social Theory)*. London & New York: Routledge.

Bako, T. & Zana, K. (2020) *Transgenerational Trauma and Therapy: The Transgenerational Atmosphere*. Abingdon, Oxon: Routledge.

Balint, M. (1979). *The Basic Fault: Therapeutic Aspects of Regression*. London & New York: Tavistock Publications.

Beaumont, H. (2012) *Toward a Spiritual Psychotherapy: Soul as a Dimension of Experience*. Berkeley, CA: North Atlantic Books.

Bollas, C. (2018) *Meaning and Melancholia: Life in the Age of Bewilderment*. Abingdon, Oxon: Routledge.

Di-Angelo, R. (2018) *White Fragility: Why It's So Hard for White People to Talk about Racism*. London: Penguin Books.

Hubl, T. (2020) *Healing Collective Trauma: A Process for Integrating Our Intergenerational and Cultural Wounds*. Boulder, CO: Sounds True.

Hughes, J.M. (1989) *Reshaping the Psycho-Analytic Domain: The Work of Melanie Klein, W.R.D. Fairbairn & D.W. Winnicott*. Berkeley & Los Angeles, CA: University of California Press.

Klein, M. (1946) Notes on some schizoid mechanisms. *The International Journal of Psychoanalysis* 1946, Vol. 27, pp. 99–110.

Racker, H. (1982) *Transference and Counter Transference*. London: Karnac.

Rogers, C.R. (1967) *On Becoming a Person: A Therapist's View of Psychotherapy*. London: Constable.

Scharmer, O. (2020) Presence, absence, and creating a holding space for trauma. In *Healing Collective Trauma: A Process for Integrating Our Intergenerational and Cultural Wounds*. Hubl, T. (Editor). Boulder, Co: Sounds True, pp. 172–178.

Sills, C. (2024) Personal Communication.

Turner, D. (2021) *Intersections of Privilege and Otherness in Counselling and Psychotherapy: Mockingbird*. Routledge: London.

Chapter 9

Carrie

Recovery of the Self

Trauma and Transcendence

I began this book by sharing with you my journey, through which my philosophy and approach as a psychotherapist emerged:

- Holding trust in the person's essence; the client as 'Thou' is a unique, individual manifestation of the divine.
- Committed to meeting and exploring their personal, transgenerational and transpersonal experiences with them, for the healing and realisation of the self, with its qualities and potential for profound personal fulfilment.

In the preceding chapters, I explored my philosophy, theory and work concerning transgenerational and complex traumas that can separate us from realising our potential as human beings. Traumas held within our body and soul are unresolved legacies from direct personal experiences and history, which cause personal alienation, existential fear and suffering. They are endured both individually and collectively. From the grim spell of such factors, which configure lives with suffering and an adaptive disconnection from self, there is a poignant question: from where do the fortitude and hope come for us to return to and persevere with the exploration of devastating histories and experiences, and to open to the immanence of our essential qualities of being, such as love, compassion, imagination and creativity? My answer is that these aspects of our essence as beings inspire us to bravely engage with horror from our past and that of our ancestors for self-realisation and a good life. As I discussed in Chapter 3, I see it as my responsibility as a psychotherapist to trust, hold and support the transcendent qualities of my clients for their reconnection with and rekindling of their personal divinity and potential.

Reflecting upon my work with Carrie, I think of her heart and spirit. Despite the terror, anxiety, toxic guilt and shame consequent of complex and transgenerational traumas, her qualities of love, courage and compassion were evident from our first meeting. They came through to me, despite her speaking in strongly self-critical ways, with punctuating offerings of the word 'sorry'. I sensed from this demeanour that she had survived an oppressive environment and history by holding both

DOI: 10.4324/9781003456438-10

a belief of being flawed and an attitude of self-blame; these being aspects of the personality style she developed for acceptance and holding within the family into which she had been born.

I felt protective towards Carrie. Through memories of my family history and childhood, I was aware of how patterned beliefs of personal fault and disclosure of non-normative experiences (*e.g.*, Unusual Subjective Experiences – USEs, as explored in Chapter 3 and reflected upon by Carrie in the Appendix) can leave us vulnerable to harm from treatments that do not appreciate and engage with the depth of our being.

However, I also appreciated that through her self-critical attitude, she conveyed a capacity for humility and self-reflection that can be of immense value if it is allied with a commitment to exploration, healing and the unfolding of the self.

Background

Carrie entered therapy with me in her late twenties, following the beginnings of recovery from a breakdown which occurred after escaping from a relationship of domestic violence and sexual abuse. An active person who was passionately engaged in her work, one morning, she woke gripped by paralysing fear, finding it difficult to rise from her bed and unable to leave her home.

She was terrified when we met for the first time, sensing the presence of her abusive ex-partner and imagining he was watching as we sat together and that he would be coming to 'get' her. Despite her terror, Carrie maintained contact with me and eloquently shared information about her background and life.

When Carrie was seven years old, her mother became ill, remaining in poor health up to the present day. From this young age, Carrie remembers becoming vigilant, deferential and responsive to her mother's emotions and wishes and pre-cociously carrying responsibility and attentiveness for the care and well-being of her two younger sisters and the family pets. I sensed this as the template for her general orientation in relationships with others. From Carrie's description of her childhood and ongoing relationship with her mother, I understood she had been ascribed in infancy the role of 'Echo' to her mother's 'Narcissus', these being names eponymously employed from the Greek myth for the concept of narcissism and its corollary, 'echoism'. Linington, Montgomery and Morris (2017) describe the effects of narcissism, which inverts the pattern of parental care into a mother and/or father's demand for attention and mirroring from their child, thus suppress-ing and sacrificing a daughter or son's development of a secure, confident self for an echoing focus upon themselves. Carrie understood from the narrative her mother bitterly emphasised and repeated, that her drive for attention and mirroring related to her relationship with her own mother during a childhood with parents who were refugees from the Holocaust.

Carrie described to me how her mother dominated their relationship with her own feelings, experiences and the competitive assertion of her needs and accom-plishments. This included exposing Carrie to intense reflections and emotions concerning the fate of the Jewish wing of the family; these were confusing and traumatising. She conveyed to me a strong resentment of her mother's behaviour and expectations and an enduring nervous holding back from asserting herself as a cumulative effect of her mother's narcissistic rage. Thus, I appreciated Carrie's attitude and demeanour which discounted the depth and value of her being, this being an issue intimately connected to her relationship with her mother.

Carrie received the modelling of a stoical attitude from her father, with the deprecation of feelings such as pain and distress. His sometimes destructive, violent anger, which she observed as directed towards her mother and sisters, was another factor in Carrie's early formation of an attitude of vigilance for the needs and care-taking of others. Thus, issues carried by both her mother and father affected Carrie towards an attentiveness for others and a discounting of her own emotions and needs. A little later in our work together, she would tell me of a desire to be 'invisible' and, on occasion, of experiencing herself as immobile and mute.

However, Carrie also told me of the redemptive, loving connection with her maternal grandfather, from whom she received the confirmation and mirroring missing from her parents. He affirmed Carrie through an undemonstrative but deeply loving conveying of acceptance, which was nourishing in her pursuit of the paths she chose that were dismissed and sometimes deprecated by her parents, such as her employment in work concerned with human rights. He also introduced Carrie to classical music, and noticing her love of the violin, he gave her one as a birthday gift. She enjoyed playing for him, seeing his quiet pleasure, including a soothing smile, when she made a mistake. I would come to appreciate the transgenerational and transformational significance of Carrie's bond with him. This was with respect to both the family's losses and travails caused by the Holocaust and its legacy, as inspirational support for her compassion towards others and her work.

As a gifted child, Carrie encountered difficult experiences in her local community and at school. She did not feel she belonged anywhere. In her early twenties, Carrie left her partner and moved to the USA for an exciting job opportunity in the field of human rights. In the small city where Carrie was located, she obtained a place in the local orchestra. She began to experience the sense of belonging she had yearned for, immersing herself in fulfilling engagement in her work. She told me of poignant 'peak experiences' (Maslow, 2011) concerning her life and self during evening walks along a footpath by the side of the local river, gazing at its flow.

However, this experience of self-actualisation challenged the introjected, self-suppressive way which had helped Carrie to traverse childhood within her family: Kalsched's 'self-care system' (2013), which I referred to in Chapters 3 and 4. Carrie began to feel guilty for 'letting down' her parents concerning their expectations of her. She also started to fear that she would ultimately fail in her work. These feelings caused her to push herself, work too hard and become distracted and disturbed by self-doubt. Around this time, her partner arrived in the USA to commence his sexual abuse of her, compounding an already established pattern of undermining, emotional abuse, which had begun in the UK.

Consistent with the negative conception of herself carried from childhood and her way of coping with hostility from her parents, she managed this horrific ordeal by discounting her feelings and their significance and being overly sympathetic to her partner's issues. In these heart-breaking circumstances, Carrie began to experience disturbing episodes of dissociation, in which she lost her sense of space and time. She could not concentrate on her violin practice or maintain her membership in the orchestra. Her trust in herself collapsed, and one day, while travelling alone on a bus, Carrie decided to leave the job she loved and return to the UK with her partner.

Following their return to the UK, he subjected Carrie to intense emotional abuse, domestic violence and rape. She tried to assert and defend herself against him, but existential terror, toxic shame and self-blame restricted these efforts. The patterns formed in childhood of self-doubt and deferential attentiveness to the feelings of others continued to dominate. In contrast to her well-developed social and political awareness, Carrie found herself believing she was 'bad', at fault and thinking that the abuse wouldn't be happening if she got things 'right' for her partner. She took despairing, often resigned, defence and refuge through freezing her responses, dissociating and hiding. Sometimes, she would try to conceal herself by shrinking into a foetal position behind a clothes airer.

Carrie's parents were unresponsive to her muted but repeated signalling of intense difficulty and distress, with her mother being focused and excited about a new phase in her own life. This was also the case with her friends, who were accustomed to her being available and attentive to their concerns and issues. In relation to such unbalanced relationships, Carrie once told me of the sense of 'sacrificing parts [of herself for others] until there is nothing left'.

After six terrible months, Carrie managed to escape from the relationship, with the ex-partner stalking her for a considerable period of time. She has shown me a photograph in which his silhouetted image can be seen from behind a curtain as she posed with friends in a café. As I'm sure you, the reader, will understand, Carrie continued to live with free-floating terror caused by her ordeal, with much of her memory closed against unbearable recollection. From within a new relationship, Carrie strove to recapture the experience of normality and a familiar sense of self. She sought to find a way back to work. However, following viewing an evocative film on television one evening, Carrie woke the morning to which I referred earlier, feeling unable to get out of bed or leave the house. The power and depth of her traumas and repressed memories had arisen to overwhelm her.

The next few months were a severe challenge for Carrie, and I felt moved by her fortitude and courage as she recounted that time to me. In addition to the feelings of terror and shame, her experience of periods of immobilisation was mystifying and profoundly worrying for her. Carrie attended counselling for a few months, and this helped her begin to recover her functioning, enabling her re-entry to employment – albeit in a basic administrative role, distant from her vocation. This was Carrie's situation at the commencement of our work together.

A Dialogue for Healing

Carrie's initial email enquiring about entering therapy with me had EMDR in the title, emphasising her need for healing from the traumas that caused her to live with intense suffering. As previously stated, it was evident to me from our early sessions that Carrie had a propensity for superfluous apologies, harsh judgement of herself, and, in addition, a driven, forensic attitude towards her personal exploration and therapy. This, I sensed, had attracted her to EMDR as a solution-focused, manualised treatment of trauma. However, I soon became concerned that we could overuse such approaches to miss her need for the experience of reparative therapeutic dialogue and contact in alignment with her cycles of experiencing. This would be repeating her experience of the relational inadequacy and neglect of Carrie's childhood environment and could reinforce the adaptation, modelled by her father to move away from feelings *via* action and work. My concern was highlighted when Carrie emphasised that our conversations were very helpful, through which we explored her traumas, current experience of life and struggles with ongoing relationships with her parents; whilst she simultaneously believed that if we didn't use EMDR in a session, she hadn't 'worked'. Through exploration, we found this attitude stemmed from doubts about her personal value. Consistent with experiences of her parents being disinterested in the depth of her being, Carrie didn't believe she was entitled to psychotherapy and compared herself to others, whose suffering she considered to be more serious and deserving of compassion. She found normatively valued, more explicitly goal-oriented approaches such as EMDR easier to justify for herself. Thus, it became clear that Carrie needed therapeutic dialogue, with my holding of an I-Thou attitude, for a healing experience of the ruptures she carried in her soul concerning her value and depth as a person.

So, our work developed through contact, exploration and dialogue, which formed the basis for our use of trauma treatments, such as EMDR and CRM, which I describe later in this chapter. I felt connected to Carrie's commitment to healing from the terror with which she lived; it resonated for me with my own long journey of processing the legacy of my family history and childhood. Her courage and sincerity were inspiring, and I felt that my early life, study and work had prepared me for this therapeutic relationship, for which fate had enabled me to be of service.

During the first year of our work together, Carrie explored with an exquisite capacity for expression and dialogue, and I was deeply affected in my heart and soul by her recounting of her ordeal of abuse. I respected the protection her psyche had provided through dissociation and a restricting of memory. In the course of our dialogues, it became evermore clear that her paralysing terror consequent of the horror was intertwined with self-blame. When we used imaginal exercises of the type I have described in Chapter 4, both aspects were evident. For example, when looking upon her traumatised self, Carrie would express judgement and frustration, with robust resistance to the compassion, which she acknowledged would naturally flow from her to someone else. From this, I sensed an intrapsychic merging of archaic material with her recent traumas.

The nightmares she brought to sessions were terrifying, unmistakable representations of the experience of mortal threat and violation perpetrated upon her by the ex-partner, as were the associated smells and images which disturbed her waking hours. She also found herself feeling compelled to avoid listening to certain pieces of classical music and watching films with specific movie stars, who she associated with her time with the ex-partner. Carrie told me of a recurring nightmare of him coming to kill her, her current partner, close friends and me, and her sense of guilt and responsibility for what befell the other people in the dream. Our exploration of the dream found it to be the expression of an intertwined, combination of traumas: sexual abuse and domestic violence, childhood trauma with introjects of responsibility and self-blame and transgenerational entanglement with the fate of the maternal wing of the family in the Holocaust. She told me that fears and nightmares of people coming to get her had been present all her life but less prominent until the trauma of her abuse.

As previously stated, Carrie needed a relational experience which affirmed and encouraged her in alliance with her keen, inquiring intellect. When she reported episodes of panic, terror and USEs, I felt care and empathy and offered reframes of her experiences as being in alignment with her therapeutic journey. For example, in response to her frightened reporting to me of a momentary experience in a shop of seeing people's faces melt, I explored with her how she had safely managed the experience and was now lucidly reflecting upon it and its significance. I offered an appreciation of this USE as a significant, healthy, albeit terrifying and disturbing arising from her unconscious, for the purpose of bringing to consciousness for healing, a compound of her traumatic experiences of others. My intention was to validate her unfolding process and encourage a self-affirming understanding of it, rather than considering herself to be unwell and so pathologising the experience. Given the intensity of the panic, terror and experiences of dissociation (in which she felt her surroundings to be unfamiliar) she suffered at times, I suggested she might wish to consult her doctor for a prescription of medication to be used if/when required for symptomatic relief. She did so, using the prescribed beta blockers thoughtfully – when needed. Carrie has recounted her reflections in the appendix of this book of crying with relief following the session when she first disclosed her USEs to me. This was in reaction to my calm, accepting and validating response to her, which contrasted with her experiences with previous therapists.

I told Carrie she could contact me between sessions if needed. This invitation challenged her patterned experience of loneliness, self-reliance and beliefs of being unworthy. Still, she responded to my additional availability when desperation overwhelmed her. These calls and extra sessions (for which I didn't charge, being aware of her low income) were spaces for holding, reassurance and connection with the safety of the present moment and the enabling of reflective, positive self-understanding. During and following episodes of panic and derealisation,

I facilitated her return to being present within her 'window of tolerance' (Ogden, Minton & Pain, 2006) with the use of the following:

- Grounding physical and observational exercises.
- Connection in here/now contact with me through conversation.
- Containment, through facilitating Carrie's visualisation of placing the unfinished business from the session into a container to be held until we next met.
- Imaginal, soul connection – to supportive figures (as discussed in Chapter 4) such as her grandfather, close friends and a female lawyer she admired.
- Carrie also possessed a pack of flashcards I purchased for her from Carolyn Spring (https://www.carolynspring.com). These flashcards have reassuring, grounding statements concerning the experience of panic and dissociation, which she kept with her to read whenever necessary.

Carrie, with her remarkable fortitude, began to accomplish a slow easing of the post-traumatic terror she carried from the abuse. In relation to our work for connection with holding and support, the loving bond with her grandfather was especially important to her. On one occasion, we used Playmobil figures for a family constellation exercise to touch her soulful connection with him and her ancestors. Following his death, we dedicated a session to honour him and his place in Carrie's life. In my therapy room, I have a special candle holder, created by a sculptor who burnished it with a tool created from an ivory handled hairbrush which originally belonged to her great grandmother, who died in Treblinka Concentration Camp. Carrie lit a tealight in it, which burned through the session.

Trust and Affirmation: Towards Reconnection with Self

As I mentioned, Carrie punctuated our conversations with superfluous apologies, which saddened me. I responded to them with reassurance and enquiry.

She frequently spoke of feeling the imminence of death, in not being able to envisage living more than a few months ahead, nor returning to her career in the field of human rights. She grieved, missing her familiar experience of self, the experiences of personal presence and belonging she had enjoyed in the USA. Carrie also lamented the dulling of her desire to pick up the violin and play each day. I believe Carrie's loss of a sense of the self that she recognised as being her was intertwined with the fracturing of her personality style, which had been overwhelmed by the abuse and its aftermath.

She didn't believe she could reconnect with or recover that self, ostensibly seeking just amelioration of the awful post-traumatic terror with which she was living. However, I sensed a residual hope from the depth of her sharing with me and her enquiring about my opinion concerning whether she could recover her Self.

Through my experience of the quality of Carrie's presence, self-awareness and commitment, I held a robust confidence in her. I articulated this in my replies to her questioning: I believed she would get through, not only to recover but, in time, blossom and flourish. I was moved from deep within me to articulate that my belief and trust in her were indestructible. I thought again of these lines concerning personal essence from 'Elements of the Real in Man: Diamond Heart Book One', which I quoted in Chapter 3:

> Essence was there in the beginning, and it is still there. Although it was not seen, not recognized, and was even rejected and hurt in many ways, it is still there. In order to protect itself, it has gone underground, under cover...
>
> (Almaas, 1987, p. 2)

On several occasions, Carrie responded to such affirmations, expressing and asserting her disbelief. I responded with support and appreciation of her candour; our engaging in this way constituted an inclusion and holding of her depth as a person.

Unfolding Path

The approach of our work together and Carrie's healing progressed, through her expression and exploration of arising feelings, memories and insights from her cycles of experiencing concerning her post-traumatic terror and deprecated self. Through our therapeutic dialogue, work within the imaginal dimension and the use of EMDR and CRM, I supported Carrie in her resolve to process the immense trauma of the abuse she had endured and survived and for the splits in her soul (Ruppert, 2007) to heal – that were expressed through terror and dissociation. She was determined to recover her sense of self-coherence and agency.

I was deeply moved and touched by Carrie in this work, which called me to collaborate closely with her commitment and perseverance in exploring fragments of her shattered and shattering experience. Carrie's memory of the six-month period in which she suffered abuse from the ex-partner was incomplete because of the self-protective dissociation which was activated for her survival. We worked with Carrie's experience of the ordeal and specific traumatic moments of paramount significance to her. These were scenes of assaults, her fierce resistance to the abuse, resignation, hiding, personal isolation and deathly resignation to fate, as well as locations, images, music and smells that activated terror and dissociation. I facilitated Carrie's expression and exploration by paying attention to her emotional and somatic experiences. From her need to exorcise her ex-partners' phantom presence from her life and reclaim her power, she had a courageous and tenacious determination towards visualising, connecting with her rage and confronting his elusive face within her mind's eye, for which EMDR and CRM were useful.

Targeted Use of EMDR and CRM

In Chapter 4, I shared my view concerning the place of manualised, protocol-driven trauma treatments in psychotherapy. I here reiterate my belief that healing occurs in their use, through love and connection between therapist and client, which provide the necessary, secure basis for a reparative experience and healing. In our work together, this was manifested by Carrie's trust in me and my deeply felt care for her as we engaged together, with her cycle of experiencing and the excruciating suffering she carried from trauma.

It was in this context that our use of CRM and EMDR aided her journey towards:

- Recovering her sense of self and personal presence.
- Undoing her retroflected anger and self-judgement concerning the abuse.
- Achieving a reconciliation and reconnection with her Self.
- Gradually triumphing over the trauma and its effects.

EMDR

I employed EMDR in the first year of Carrie's therapy to support her towards facing and managing the horrific effects of the ex-partner's abuse of her, and here I outline some of the key elements of our work with EMDR. This is not an exhaustive summary of my use of EMDR with Carrie. For further information about EMDR, I recommend Shapiro (2001), Parnell (2007), and Forgash and Copeley (2008).

- Use of the 'Back of Head' scale (Knipe, 2008). This is a safety aid to help us monitor levels of personal presence and dissociation before, during and after work with traumatic memories. I would ask Carrie to imagine a line from the edge of her forehead to the back of her head: The position at the edge of her forehead represented her being fully present, whilst the position at the back of her head indicated her being seriously dissociation by the memory and image of the trauma with which we were working. I periodically asked Carrie to place her hand against her head to measure and indicate her level of presence and dissociation throughout the process.
- Gentle pendulation between safety and an image of the ex-partner. This technique is also drawn from Knipe's work (2008), which enables a movement between the present moment and the trauma. Carrie would look at a photograph she liked of my cat, Corky, on the wall behind me and in front of her. This pleasant experience was reinforced by her following my hand with eyes, moving back and forth a few times from left to right, for horizontal 'bilateral stimulation', an intrinsic part of EMDR (Shapiro, 2001). Then, I would ask Carrie to bring to mind for five seconds the image of the trauma she had chosen to work with and then return to looking at Corky with more bilateral stimulation. Gradually, Carrie was able to tolerate the holding of the traumatic image in her mind's eye for longer, eventually with my adding bilateral stimulation to support processing the trauma.
- In time, we progressed to using the standard EMDR protocol (Shapiro, 2001) to engage with the selected memories and images she was drawn to processing.
- Carrie's sensing of supportive figures with and behind her aided this work, as did the container exercise I described earlier. At the end of the session, after

grounding exercises, and the pleasant place procedure I referred to in Chapter 4, I would help her to reflect on a positive perspective to which she had access, asking her to find and bring up a representative, pleasant image of it in her mind's eye, *e.g.*, visiting her current partner's home country, with him. I would apply several sets of vertical bilateral stimulation to reinforce its positive effects until she reached a plateau in this experience.

CRM

The intensity of Carrie's fear and distress in this work led me to introduce the use of CRM (Schwarz, Corrigan, Hull & Raju, 2017) with its integral, multi-layered imaginal holding for trauma processing. Again, for clarity and the purpose of this chapter, I offer a simplified summary.

I facilitated:

1 Breathwork to help Carrie relax and become open to engaging with the scene from the trauma she had chosen to work with on each occasion.

   Throughout this process, I would offer different breathing exercises (as described in Schwarz, Corrigan, Hull & Raju, 2017) appropriate to the different phases of the work, such as those that could help her feel personal power, discharge feelings or feel grounded.

2 Carrie's construction, visualising and forming a 'resource grid' (Schwarz, Corrigan, Hull & Raju, 2017, pp. 96–109), within which she felt held, with an orientation of herself within the grid through the setting of an 'eye position' (Schwarz, Corrigan, Hull & Raju, 2017, p. 48).

3 Visualisation of herself at the age when her ex-partner abused her and then imagine a soothing figure of her choice (*e.g.*, a loving, faithful dog) to come into view for that part to cuddle.

4 Carrie's observing self to visualise, contact and experience holding and support from a reassuring mentor figure, such as a female lawyer she admired. This was to introduce additional support for her bearing of the painful sight of her younger self, who, in appearance and demeanour, wore the effects of her abuse.

5 Eye contact and shared breathing between her observing and younger self – these were important for her sense of inner cohesion and the support of her younger self.

6 With the layers of holding I have described in place, we confronted, through visualisation, sensing and our dialogue, the memory of the abuse, with the purposes I have listed above that were crucial for Carrie.

7 Carrie was determined to become visually present to herself in the scene of abuse and to confront the face of her ex-partner – this constituted her regaining of power and agency. It required several sessions, culminating with (alongside my affirming of its significance and a reassuring discussion, differentiating the therapeutic use of imagination from actual, physical behaviour) a releasing expression of rage through her visualising killing him by driving a car over him.

8   The facilitation in these sessions through visualisation and dialogue, of contact between her two parts involved in the work – a movement towards a healing rapprochement with her younger self and an easing of self-blame and judgement.

On several occasions, we needed to end the CRM session early (*i.e.,* before Carrie's settling, relaxing and reflecting within the visualised and sense experience of a sacred or pleasant scene), her being overwhelmingly distressed and/or frightened. I supported her in the ways I have described earlier. I believe these were ultimately positive moments of reparative contact through the confirming and affirming care of our conversations, with my availability for follow-up calls and extra sessions.

Progress Beyond Trauma Treatment Protocols

Eventually, we settled into working without EMDR, CRM or DBR (which we tried but didn't suit her), with our dialogue and flexible use of the imaginal dimension for Carrie to express, explore and process her phenomenological, gestalt cycle of experiencing which took place in and between sessions. This attention to her process, without the imposition of a treatment protocol, relieved Carrie of the additional pressure and intensity that she had experienced through the use of EMDR and CRM. The therapy progressed as she expressed, confronted and processed memories of abuse, supported by grounding exercises, reflection and consolidation within the here/now. The care I felt and expressed to her was, I believe, a reparative and moving experience for her, which contrasted with the hate she had suffered from the ex-partner in his attacks on her and also the disinterest of her parents at times of desperate need.

The connection and contact between us were especially crucial when memories of traumas burst into feeling and consciousness with shocking, terrifying intensity, such as – when her ex-partner pushed and assaulted her against a wardrobe – feeling she was going to die; sexual assault; rape; hiding from him in the bathroom. Thus, our work unfolded through Carrie's courage, commitment and the strength of our therapeutic relationship.

Carrie's commitment within sessions was mirrored in her engagement with life outside the therapy room. Despite setbacks, including intense personal hardship during the COVID pandemic and lockdown, she moved forward, with a reduction in the frequency and intensity of experiences of post-traumatic terror. Carrie found a new job to resume her career and contribution to the field of human rights, and this success was an indication of her healing and progress. She formed a relationship of love and respect with a new partner. In addition, she happily returned to playing her violin and joined a chamber orchestra based in her locality. With these advances, Carrie's personality style of being 'Echo' to her mother and others receded, with deepening awareness and assertion of her rights and wishes. She became more assertive in holding her boundaries towards her mother's expectations and demands for attention. In expanding appreciation of her personal value, needs and desires, Carrie moved away from unbalanced friendships and acquaintances, forming new and more nourishing ones.

Carrie experienced her progress as the cause of a catalytic dissonance, between the confirmation of her value and qualities and her negative beliefs about herself and the world. Her professional accomplishments and affirmations from managers and colleagues were highly significant factors in activating feelings of shame, bewilderment and episodes of dissociation. I understood this aspect of Carrie's process to be the symptomatic manifestation of effects from her cumulative and complex traumas, these being a transgenerational entanglement with the Holocaust, experiences of childhood neglect as 'Echo' to her mother and sexual and domestic violence. They are the roots of her negative and inaccurate beliefs about herself and an old adaptive, protective pattern of self-effacement towards those she admires and who carry authority. As before, I utilised our therapeutic alliance for holding and support of Carrie's exploration, processing and healing from this legacy of her traumas.

Although less frequently, Carrie continued to follow my invitation to contact me between sessions when a sense of overwhelm and/or dissociation occurred. The additional support I provided to Carrie in these conversations and supplementary sessions aided her persistence and consolidation of progress along her unfolding path and provided protection from a re-traumatisation, which can result from a lonely enduring of returning memories.

Summary

In the past two years, Carrie's healing from the effects of trauma has continued with a very significant reduction in their intensity. The progress of her life has continued to unfold. She has achieved dramatic advances in her career and is more trusting and assertive of her needs and rights in both her work and relationships. Her accomplishments reflect her personal value, have increased her visibility and garnered affirmations from managers and senior colleagues. We have continued to work together on the challenging effects of such positive experiences, which I referred to just a little earlier, and she is steadily becoming more comfortable with her relationships with colleagues, her personal authority and her accomplishments.

In Chapter 4, I discussed the Jungian concept of the interactive field, which can hold transference in broad and non-hierarchical ways and have reflected on this with respect to my work with Carrie. As I have previously stated, I believe there has been a profound interaction between us. Our respective histories and personal journeys have impacted upon each other. Her struggle, fortitude and commitment to healing, along with her relationship to the Holocaust through her maternal line and crucial connection with her grandfather, have touched my history and journey of reconnection with my essential self, inspiring and energising my care for her unfolding process. In our work together, I have felt the presence of my ancestors, as she has her grandfather.

Carrie still conveys a transference from her relationships with her parents, manifested in superfluous apologies and feelings of being unentitled and guilty about receiving my support and that from her senior colleagues. We continue to explore this together, with awareness of her inherent personal power, which she is progressively experiencing and expressing through her dreams, beliefs and actions.

She has said that when first entering therapy with me, she thought she hated men, particularly those in authority. Given the depth of her sharing and strong engagement with me from the start of our work together, I have found this to be an extraordinary disclosure. My understanding is that there has been and is a serendipitous interaction between us that has allowed her, despite her damaging experiences with men, to be courageously open with me; and for me to maintain an unbreakable trust in her throughout and during her darkest and most terrifying moments. She has told me, 'I had never met a man like you before' and 'It wasn't just that I didn't think I could do those things anymore; I was gone…you brought me back'. I never thought she was 'gone', and the success of our work together reflects the strength of the therapeutic relationship we swiftly formed in her first session.

At times, in a parallel process with Carrie's, I have doubted myself and my abilities and been troubled by toxic shame from the traumas of my own family history and childhood, the story and legacy of which I shared in the first chapter of this book. I am very grateful to Peter Orlandi-Fantini, my clinical supervisor, who provided me with holding and loving support with respect to those resonances and activations from my own suffering.

Throughout our work together, I have appreciated Carrie's depth as a person and her living with several forms and layers of trauma. I feel privileged to be a collaborator and a companion with her on her path of fortitude and heart. With significant parallels to my own background, working with Carrie has been a rewarding and healing experience for me, through the opportunity to hold and affirm her value as a human being and help her in ways that were impossible for me to do for my childhood family and ancestors.

References

Almaas, A.H. (1987) *Diamond Heart, Book 1: Elements of the Real in Man.* Boston, MA: Shambhala.

Forgash, C. & Copeley, M. (2008, Editors). *Healing the Heart of Trauma and Dissociation with EMDR and Ego State Therapy.* New York: Springer, pp. 181–217.

Kalsched, D. (2013) *Trauma and the Soul: A Psycho-Spiritual Approach to Human Development and Its Interruption.* London & New York: Routledge.

Knipe, J. (2008) Loving eyes: Procedures to therapeutically reverse dissociative processes while preserving emotional safety. In *Healing the Heart of Trauma and Dissociation with EMDR and Ego State Therapy.* Forgash, C. & Copeley, M. (Editors). New York: Springer, pp. 181–217.

Linington, M., Montgomery, N. & Morris, E. (2017) Echoism: A life dominated by concern for the other. In: *ATTACHMENT: New Directions in Psychotherapy and Relational Psychoanalysis* July 2017, Vol. 11, pp. 134–153.

Maslow, A. H. (2011) *Toward a Psychology of Being.* Blacksburg, VA: Wilder Publications, Inc.

Ogden, P., Minton, K. & Pain, K. (2006) *Trauma and the Body: A Sensorimotor Approach to Psychotherapy.* New York: Norton.

Parnell, L. (2007) *A Therapist's Guide to EMDR: Tools and Techniques for Successful Treatment.* New York & London: Norton.

Ruppert, F. (2007) *Splits in the Soul: Integrating Traumatic Experiences.* West Sussex: Green Balloon Publishing.

Schwarz, L., Corrigan, F., Hull, A. & Raju, R. (2017) *Explorations in Mental Health 17: The Comprehensive Resource Model: Effective Therapeutic Techniques for the Healing of Complex Trauma.* Abingdon, Oxon: Routledge.

Shapiro, F. (2001) *Eye Movement Desensitization and Reprocessing: Basic Principles, Protocols, and Procedures*, Second Edition. New York: Guildford.

Concluding Thoughts

I was born into a devastated and traumatised family, which inspired me towards a life of reflection and healing, the work of soul-based psychotherapy, and to write this book.

The alienated, shadow side of our human condition is apparent in the worn, torn and warring world in which we live. Recognising one's own lostness in the madness and tragedies portrayed in the news can be salutary, and such awareness can catalyse us to connect with another way of being.

I believe in our ultimate spiritual unity and depth, which transcends space and time, and from which, with love, trust and practices such as psychotherapy, movements of profound healing can occur; for us to live with fulfilment and relate to others with care, understanding and appreciation of our connectedness and diversity. Instead of being transfixed with fear and hate by shadows of our suffering which we cast upon others, we need to be conscious and attentive to our own woundedness and flaws. It is for this purpose my approach to complex and transgenerational trauma is dedicated, with the following key elements:

- Holding the self with compassion and respect as an individual and unique manifestation from the spiritual ground of being.
- Meeting clients with an I-Thou attitude towards them and their potential for healing and personal unfolding.
- Attending to the effects of complex and transgenerational trauma with an integrative, phenomenological method and approach, which has been drawn and adapted from gestalt therapy.
- Inclusion of the transgenerational as an integral aspect of trauma therapy and psychotherapy.

I am very grateful to all the clients about whom I have written. I feel privileged to be/have been their therapist, and I deeply appreciate their reading and vital feedback concerning the case studies and vignettes of our work together. I feel blessed to have/have had the opportunity to be of service to people who are alive now, and this, I acknowledge with gratitude, has provided healing for my soul and perhaps of my ancestors, too.

DOI: 10.4324/9781003456438-11

Clients' Reflections

I here gratefully include contributions from clients who have appeared in this book, each with a distinctive voice.

Here Are Robert's Reflections on the Event Described in Chapter 1

In 2013, I was in my third year of studies for a BSc (Hons) degree in counselling and integrative psychotherapy. To complete my studies, I was required to undertake 240 hours of personal therapy. Tuesday morning at 10.00 was my regular appointment time for therapy with Isaac.

The sessions always started with a cup tea, although on this occasion the kettle needed to be replenished with water. As Isaac left to do so, I started to peruse the room, his certificates, the titles on the bookshelf, the pictures displayed. I was drawn by one picture, a slightly faded black and white family grouping which I assumed was taken early in the twentieth century.

I knew Isaac was of Jewish descent, and as I immersed my feelings in this picture, the word 'Holocaust' filled my thoughts and my emotions, why? I had recently been though my own personal holocaust, an acrimonious divorce which culminated in me losing all contact with my daughter; my family. Did I handle the picture? No, I did not touch or handle it. I intensely viewed it, with my thoughts being to its meaning for self and others.

Isaac returned, and with the tea made, the session started. I commented and then inquired about the picture, Isaac confirmed, indeed the picture was of his relatives, many which had perished in the concentration camps during the Second World war. In response, I uttered the word 'family' and with that utterance the picture fell and smashed on the floor, both myself and Isaac where now on our knees, stunned by this phenomenal event.

Reflection/Interpretation

The use of self-disclosure by therapists has been debated by many schools, for its use, my professional stance as a therapist carries two caveats: Firstly, my disclosure will do no harm; thus, it will contribute to the client's process, and secondly, it is not for my own professional or personal gain or gratification. Furthermore, I am not reliant on coincidence; my sense is that all events occur within a personal or greater global arena as an opportunity for me and others (humanity) to evolve.

However, when reflecting upon the moment the picture fell. I recall how the sound of shattering glass impacted my senses, then, my realisation that it was Isaac's family picture, which for me immortalised pictorial and symbolic relational content, which now may have been irrevocably damaged.

Here, I need to state as a trainee therapist one attends personal therapy with an emerging knowledge of the therapeutic relationship, and its processional endeavours for both personal growth and ongoing professional development.

Thus far I have attempted to set the scene by recalling a past narrative, whereas now I consider my current understanding. As I have stated before I do not adhere to coincidences. So how do I explain, understand and give meaning to, and for, the event. My answer is I do not know, what I do know is that the event was curiously cathartic. Therefore my synopsis is as follows:

> *I was in the presence of a significate other (my therapist) whom I had built a trusted relationship with. I fundamentally was in his space that he was willing to share with me, a space which displayed his nature whilst being imbued by his essence. In person he carried within himself his own experience of life thus far and his acquired academic knowledge, also second generational knowledge and a genealogical blueprint from the past that encompass humanity's successes and failures.*
>
> *I know of no reason why universal forces would not intervene. My therapist had chosen to share and display much, including his family photo, it was not hidden, and in as such, these people were in the room, pictorially visible and present within a conduit of genetically transferred DNA, cell structure, and an unfolding soul.*
>
> *I cannot define why the picture fell from the wall, although in reflection when on my knees with my therapist alongside me, I was now not alone with my pain; there was a mutual connectedness through our joint loss, which facilitated a greater understanding and appreciation for my personal situation.*
> *Robert.*

Lily, Who We Met in Chapters 5 and 7 Has Composed and Shares These Lines with Us

From Bound to Bond

> *I never knew the seeds that my ancestors had sown, until I knew; I realise now that I have always known!*
> *I am all that came before me and much more.*
> *I am with them and I am free from them, I no longer run and hide.*

I wouldn't change the darkest moments, for they have brought me here.
I can live fully whilst knowing the pain of my history.
Amidst the dark days, I can hold light.
I now live in tune with my heart and my soul, and for that I am eternally grateful.
From bound to bond, thanks to you!
Back to My Essence
And now I write! I write and write and write and write and I love it. I can't believe it's taken me over 40 years to find passion! Yet I'm glad it's taken me this long, it's been 40 years in the making. I don't take it for granted, and I needed to overcome many challenges first. I love my craft and my work – I am blessed. I look forward to the many more mysteries that lie in my path ahead; I'll take the bad with the good!
Lily.

I Described My Work with Rose in Chapter 7, Here Are Her Reflections

My families came through their world wars intact, apart from my grandfather's foot which he left in the Somme in 1916. Nobody died, so we were lucky. An aunt in one family was a godmother for the other, but my parents didn't know that before they met. They were each the first in their family to go to university, where they fell in love and discovered the connection between their families. That also felt like luck. We were a lucky, happy family. That was our story, regularly told and re-told. It is, as always, not the whole story. Yes, my families were more or less physically intact. But emotionally and mentally, they were a mess.

The feeling I had no name for was a shaking, trembling feeling, like an internal earthquake. Not frequent, but powerful and recognisable. The first time it happened I was around eight years old, it was bedtime and my parents were worried; they called the doctor. After that the shaking usually came later at night and only occasionally at other times, when it was difficult to suppress, but I managed, being a mistress of the art of suppressing my feelings. At night, I would lie in my bed enduring whole-body shivers, my arms and legs twitching and juddering, wondering what was wrong with me. Eventually it would stop and I could sleep. I was so relieved when Isaac explained that this experience was my body releasing trauma at a time and in a place where I felt safe to do so. This meant I could reframe it as a positive experience and not a terrifying mysterious neurological disease.

A lot of my work with Isaac involved reframing my experiences. My autism diagnosis was the biggest reframe of all, and I am sure it landed so well with me because of all the preparatory reframing I had done with Isaac. Though when I began working with Isaac, neither of us had any idea I might be autistic; that came later, so to some extent I may also be reframing the work we did together. But when I received my diagnosis, although I knew that logically this was not the case, I really felt as though it was what I had been working towards with Isaac.

And perhaps, in a way, it was, because the two elements – the work I had done with Isaac, and my diagnosis – combined in me to create a sense of wholeness.

I had done therapeutic work before, with other good therapists, and it all helped, but without the diagnosis I don't think I would ever have got all the way to where I needed to be. Yet diagnosis isn't always such a positive experience. Some late-diagnosed autistic women experience identity crises, impostor syndrome, relationship conflicts and other difficulties as a result of their diagnosis. I experienced a great relief and joy, as parts of me that had never made sense to myself suddenly had a place in my being. I think if I had not done the work I did with Isaac over the preceding couple of years, or if my family and friends had not been supportive, my experience might have been very different. So now, for real, I feel lucky and happy.

Rose.

Here Are Reflections from Carrie for Whom Chapter 9 Is Dedicated

During Autumn 2018, I began to have unusual subjective experiences, firstly as the impression during a seminar at university that the faces of my colleagues and peers were melting, and subsequently as sightings of people, faces or still objects such as words or food moving. These experiences were terrifying and largely seemed disconnected in content and time, and having experienced what I would term a nervous breakdown a few years earlier, were compounded by the fact that I thought that I may be irretrievably losing my mind. Having left an intimate partner relationship where I was subject to repeated sexual, emotional and physical abuse, and having navigated other distressing life experiences without these sightings occurring made finding a meaning in them difficult. I had (and sometimes still have) difficulty understanding how I was seemingly able to cope with certain life events without these unusual subjective experiences, and then suddenly they seemed to occur in a way that I did not see as immediately predictable.

They brought to mind Kristeva's (1982, p. 1) description of part of abjection as 'one of those violent, dark revolts of being, directed against a threat that seems to emanate from an exorbitant outside or inside, ejected beyond the scope of the possible, the tolerable, the thinkable', and the confusion I felt with those initial experiences really did feel like a revolt of being which was 'violent' and directed against a non-specific threat, which I was unsure of the location of (and I mean this in the most figurative way possible). Though in the years since these started they have gradually started to disappear, and I hope that one day they will stop permanently, I feel very fortunate to have been able to open up to several understanding close friends and superiors at work about the experiences which has really helped to reduce their power, and to validate them as an expression of something rather than as a grave deficit in my mind, which is how I first saw them.

Having had what I would term 'a breakdown' several years before and receiving medical care which, though I felt it was often coming from a good place and was not lacking in empathy on many occasions, involved the prescription of sedatives or antidepressants and long waits for limited sessions of cognitive behavioural therapy which I feel aggravated the issues without resolving them, I was fearful of seeking help on this issue, and concerned that my therapist would suggest I go to A and E, medicate myself (which is something I have done if necessary, but only through choice), or worse, become panicked and upset at what I was experiencing. I distinctly remember crying in relief on the bus that I was actually able to take home after calling my therapist on this first instance, as none of the above happened. Though I don't remember a huge amount of what was said, I remember I had hidden myself on the floor of a toilet cubicle, terrified, and that a huge amount of time, care and patience was taken helping me to leave that cubicle and go outside of the building I was in. I remember having the awareness that what was happening and what I was seeing wasn't what other people were seeing and wasn't a continuous state, but the paranoia and terror I felt were very real indeed.

I think it has been really important that the things that I have seen subsequently have been far more ordinary – a beetle, a person sitting on a branch in a tree, a person moving in a still photograph. I currently don't regularly experience these USEs, but I feel confident that should this happen again, I would be better prepared and supported for dealing with them and would eventually be able to find some sense in the experiences themselves. I love films, and some of the earlier more terrifying things I saw were characters (often male, often fluid in shape and colour) from films I had seen, which I have been unable to re-watch because of these experiences. Instead of denying my anger at this, and the choice of film that I feel my prior subjection to violence and aggression had removed from my life, on several occasions, I have explored this anger and resentment in therapy at the fear that I would see something which would connect with my trauma, and I am increasingly able to express anger in a way that feels safe, something entirely new to me and which I really value as an experience.

I have no doubt that without therapy I would have struggled to find meaning for these experiences. Though I am often frustrated and exhausted by my own processes, and I have thought many times about avoiding appointments or certain issues, I recognise that these USEs, though terrifying and deeply uncomfortable, were also profound and have enabled me in the long term to speak about my feelings, and how these manifest in a way that would not have previously been possible. In my employment, I have assisted and continue to assist people experiencing realities different to mine, and experiencing this for myself has made me calmer, more empathetic and ultimately more reflective and better equipped in the way I do this. Though at times it is difficult, I'm glad I approached this type of therapy at a relatively young age, as it has allowed me to put the experiences and the feelings which were outside of the tolerable (Kristeva, 1982, p. 1) back into words, and to use this process and the experience of USEs to help me learn to navigate the everyday, with the very generous support of my therapist, in a way that is my own choice.

Reference

Kristeva, J. (1982) *Powers of Horror: An Essay on Abjection* (trans. L. S. Roudiez). New York: Columbia University Press.

Index

Note: *Italic* page numbers refer to figures.

Abraham, Karl 26
Activating Stimulus (AS) 58
aid therapy 64
alchemical attitude 3
Alejandra (case study) 118–120
Almaas, A.H. 1–2, 22, 24, 37–41, 72
Angela (case study) 50; agoraphobia
    78–79; complex trauma 76; DBR 84;
    ego-state therapy 80; gender dysphoria
    77; gestalt cycles of experience 79; hold
    and support 82–83; home rules 77–78;
    psyche 80–82, *81–83*; reflections 85–86;
    self-care system 80; self-starvation 81;
    transgenerational dimension 84
anti-black racism 122
Anti-Judaism 26
antisemitic oppression 11–12
antisemitism 18, 25–27, 29, 113, 118–119,
    121
Aron, L. 27
Aronson, S. 32
Assagioli, R. 19, 20, 32
Atkinson, J. 87
attentional violence 123
authentic self 21

Baehr, P. 120, 122
Bako, T. 4, 89, 104, 116, 122
Barrie, J.M. 71
Beaumont, H. 92, 93, 95, 115, 117,
    120–121
Berne, Eric 32
Bill (case study) 65, 102
Bion, Wilfred 28
blind love 91
Bollas, C. 3, 41, 60, 123, 124

Bowyer, Frank 13–14
Brickman, C. 27
Broughton, V. 92
Brown, R.S. 2, 37, 38, 52
Buber, M. 1, 23, 31, 36, 37, 39, 48

Carrie (case study) 3, 20, 45, 56, 57,
    123, 146–147; CRM 137–138;
    DBR 138; echoism 129, 138, 139;
    EMDR 136–138; healing 132–134;
    narcissism 129; resource grid 137;
    self-actualisation 130; self-realisation
    128; transcendence 128–129; trauma
    128–129, 133, 140; trust and affirmation
    134–135; window of tolerance 133–134
Caruth, C. 88
Catherine (case study) 100–102
Christie-Sands, J. 59
collective trauma 2, 87, 104, 115, 116, 120
collective unconscious 60, 61
complex trauma 1–3, 21, 36, 44–46, 60, 67,
    76, 80, 120, 128, 139, 142
compound trauma 57–58
comprehensive resource model (CRM) 56,
    63, 132, 135–138
concordant countertransference 60
consciousness 20, 56–57, 87
Copeley, M. 136
Corrigan, F.M. 58, 59, 63
cumulative oppression 123
cumulative trauma 57–58
Cushman, P. 27, 28

Davoine, F. 55, 86, 88, 91
deep brain reorienting (DBR) 56, 58–59,
    138

depressive position 117
diamond approach 22
Di-Angelo, R. 115, 122
Diller, J.V. 26
dissociation 50, 55, 57, 58, 60, 80, 119,
   121, 131–136, 139
dual awareness, therapeutic 57
Dylan, Bob 5, 13
dynamic-dialectical model 20–21

Eastwood, Clint 80
echoism 129, 138, 139
ego-state therapy 80
Emily (case study) 21, 61; first phase of
   therapy 72–73; second phase of therapy
   73; transcendent creative self 71; trauma
   73–74; writing and progress 74–75
enlightened love 91, 92
entanglement/s 1, 12–13, 43, 44, 54, 57, 61,
   88, 90–94, 97, 98, 100, 102, 107, 109,
   133, 139
Erskine, R. 57
The Essential Self 6, 37, 53, 139
Esterson, A. 13
Evans, Ken 26, 89
eye movement desensitisation and
   reprocessing (EMDR) 56, 62, 132,
   136–138

family 14, 14–15; renewal 15, 15
family constellations 6, 9, 12, 22, 74, 84,
   89, 101, 125; blind and enlightened
   love 91–92; floor tiles 94; playmobil
   figures 94; soulful connection 93–94;
   transgenerational 90–91; visualisation
   94; workshop 92–93
Ferrer, J.N. 23, 24
Forgash, C. 136
Frank, Anne 32
Freud, Sigmund 2, 26–32
Friedman, M. 23
Fromm, E. 31–32
Frosh, S. 26, 29–30
fundamental narcissism 41–42

Gaudilliere, G.M. 55, 86, 88, 91
gender dysphoria 77
Gestalt therapy 2, 13, 32, 56–61, 70, 73,
   79, 80, 85, 86, 95, 97, 99, 111, 120, 138,
   142; creative adjustment 50; cycle of
   experience 49, 51, 54; I-Thou and I-It
   48, 50; and self 48, 51–54; and trauma
   48–51; unfinished business 49

Grof, C. 45
Grof, S. 45

Hamburger, A. 88
Handelman, S.A. 30
Hartelius, G. 23
healing 43–46, 54–65, 70–71, 108–112,
   124, 128, 132–134, 139
heart: awareness 64; desires 64–65, 92
Hellinger, B. 44, 90
Hemming, Judith 12
Hermann, J. 32, 58
Hillman, J. 90, 111
House, R. 45
Howell, E.F. 57
Hubl, T. 116
Hull, A. 63
humanistic psychotherapy 18, 23–25,
   31–32
Huxley, A. 20
Hycner, R. 23, 53

identity politics 117
I-It 36, 40, 43, 48
imaginal dimension 61, 64, 69, 94, 98, 107,
   109, 135, 138
instrumental self 21
internalised transgenerational wounds 119
intersectional theory 115, 117–121
I-Thou 1, 6, 23, 36, 38–40, 43, 48, 50, 86,
   118, 126, 128, 132, 142

Jacobs, L. 23, 48
Janet, Pierre 57, 58
Jennings, J. 30
Jewish journey 24–32
Jewish science 26
Jung, C.G. 37–38, 45, 61, 90

Kalsched, D. 44, 50, 80, 130
Kampenhout, D.V. 91
Kearney, B.E. 58
Keats, John 43
Kernberg, Otto 31
Klein, D.B. 27, 29–31
Klein, M. 116–117
Knipe, J. 63, 136
Kohut, Heinz 31
Kristeva, J. 146

Laing, R.D. 13
Lancaster, B.L. 25
Laub, D. 88

Levine, P.A. 32, 51
Lily (case study) 21, 43, 49–50, 61, 95,
    97–98, 144–145; healing 70–71;
    motherhood 70–71; psychotherapy
    68; 'the missing piece' 69, 71;
    transgenerational dynamics 67; trauma
    68–69
Lings, M. 19
Linington, M. 129

Mahler, Margaret 31
Maslow, A.H. 32, 39
Mate, G. 33
McQueen, Steve 80
mental illness 13
mentalization 60
Michael (case study) 91, 95, 102; COVID
    pandemic 103, 106, 108, 111; medical
    procedures 107; overprotective 104;
    relationship 104–105; release and
    relaxation 105; self healing 111–112;
    suitcase for healing 108–111;
    transgenerational trauma 107–108;
    Ukraine War 106–107; Zoom work 103
microaggression 118
Miller, J.C. 37, 38
Minnaur, C. 19
Montgomery, N. 129
Morgan, Sian 63
Morris, E. 129

Naranjo, C. 52
narcissism 23, 41, 122, 129
negative paranoia 124–125
neuroscience-based approach 61
Nirenberg, D. 26

object relations, psychoanalytic
    psychotherapy 114
Orienting Tension (OT) 59
Orlandi-Fantini, Peter 140

paranoid schizoid position 116–117
Parlett, M. 52–53
Parnell, L. 136
participatory theory 18, 20, 23–25
perennial philosophy 19–20, 23, 24
Perls, F. 32, 49, 51, 57
Perls, Laura 32
personal awareness 64
personal consciousness 21
personality 22, 37–40, 44, 72, 119, 120,
    129, 134, 138

personal truth 42–43
Philippson, P. 51–53
Porges, S. 33, 58
positive paranoia 124
pre-personal consciousness 20
psychoanalysis 2, 18, 25–32
psychodynamic process 118
psychotherapy 1, 6, 9, 13, 16, 36–38,
    54, 68, 76, 93, 121, 132, 135, 143;
    experiencing self 40; gestalt therapy
    48, 85; intersectional theory 115,
    117–118, 120; I-Thou and I-It 43;
    Jewish journey 24–32; job of 42;
    personal resilience 89; self 41, 53, 97;
    soul 142; therapeutic alliance 123;
    training 89; transgenerational dimension
    87–89, 97, 115–116; transpersonal 2,
    18–24, 40, 114

Raju, R. 63
Robert (vignette) 14–15, 143–144
Rogers, C.R. 37, 120
Rose (case study) 98–100, 145–146
Rothschild, B. 32
Rowan, J. 10, 18–19, 21, 39–41, 52, 61,
    114
Ruppert, F. 50–51, 59–60

Sabine (case study) 22, 125–126
Salonika 4–6, 11, 110
Sardello, R. 61, 64
Schneider, J.R. 91
Schwartz, H. 26, 27
Schwartz-Salant, N. 3
Schwarz, L. 63
self 1–3, 14, 19, 20, 24, 28–29, 63,
    71–74, 79–82, 98–103, 106, 108–110,
    116–124, 142, 143; actualization
    32; and alienation 41–42; authentic
    21; care system 130; commencing
    therapy 68; consciousness 87; CRM
    137–138; EMDR 136–137; Essential
    6; experiencing self 40–41; family
    constellations 90–94; gestalt therapy
    48, 49, 51–54; healing 43–46, 111–112,
    132–134, 139; immobilisation 131;
    instrumental 21; and personality
    37–40; protective defences 64–65,
    85–86; qualities 54, 55, 60, 62;
    transcendence 128–129; transpersonal
    21; trauma 50, 128–129; trust and
    affirmation 134–135; undercover 22;
    writing 74–75

self-actualisation 39
self-care system 45, 50, 80, 130
self-realisation 1, 14, 36, 37, 39, 43–46,
    128
Shapiro, F. 32, 136
Sheldrake, R. 92
Socialist Party of Great Britain 10
soul 1–3, 7–11, 14, 15, 18, 20, 21,
    27–28, 44, 71, 73, 76, 109, 132,
    134; collective 89, 90; commencing
    therapy 68; development 38; family
    constellations 90–94; I-Thou 36, 38,
    132; Jewish journey 24; psychotherapy
    24, 142; reflections 85; self-protective
    defences 64–65; splits 59–60, 135;
    transgenerational 95, 107, 115, 116, 120;
    transpersonal self 21; trauma 41, 55, 57,
    59, 105, 121, 128; unity 115
spiritual emergency 45
spiritual retreats: family constellation
    6; May 2014 6–7; May 2015 7–9;
    transgenerational trauma 6
Starr, K. 28, 29
structural hierarchical model 21–22
Symington, N. 41, 42

therapeutic alliance 123, 125, 139
therapeutic contact & relationship 36–37,
    39, 42, 43, 45–46, 48, 52, 57, 62, 120,
    132, 138, 140, 144
therapeutic process 2, 3, 37, 58, 60, 79, 97,
    105, 109
therapeutic relationship see therapeutic
    contact & relationship
toxic shame 64–65
transgenerational 7, 16, 22, 40, 70, 84, 105,
    130; anti-black racism 122; antisemitism
    113; atmosphere 4, 13, 104, 116;
    entanglements 100, 133, 139; family
    constellations 90–94; gestalt therapy 53;
    healing 110, 128; internalised wounds
    119; interpersonal process 54;
    medical procedures 107; psychotherapy
    87–89, 97, 115–116; self 43, 65;
    soul-based systemic work 95;
    synchronistic events 61; see also
    transgenerational trauma

transgenerational trauma 1, 3, 6, 12, 13, 18,
    22, 36, 42, 60, 61, 87, 95, 98, 107–108,
    113, 115–121, 128, 142
transpersonal dimension 1, 2, 16,
    38, 39, 65, 88, 90, 110, 115, 120,
    121, 128; diamond approach 22;
    dynamic-dialectical model 20–21;
    experiencing self 40; gestalt therapy 53,
    54; healing 43, 54–65; Jewish journey
    24, 30, 32; legacy and bequest 24–25;
    participatory theory 23–25; perennial
    philosophy 19–20; personal 21;
    pre-personal 20; psychotherapy 18–19,
    24, 114, 135–136; secular conception
    51; spiritual 52–54; structural
    hierarchical model 21–22; synchronistic
    events 61
trauma 1–3, 16, 20, 32, 37–40, 67–69, 71,
    73, 74, 85, 91–92, 97, 101, 104, 107,
    110, 113–114, 140, 145, 147; CRM 137,
    138; EMDR 136–138; entanglement
    93, 95; gestalt therapy 48–54; group
    identifications 121–122; healing
    43–45, 124, 132–134; identity and
    object relations 114–115; intersectional
    theory 117–121; self 41–43, 51–54;
    and transcendence 128–129; see also
    individual entries
trauma therapy 22, 32, 50–51, 54, 55, 57,
    58, 117–121, 142
tribal soul 91–92
Turner, D. 115, 117–120

unity consciousness 20
universal soul 91–92
Unusual Subjective Experience (USE) 45

Walsby, Harold 10
Washburn, Michael 20–22, 24
White privilege 122
Wilber, K. 19, 21–22, 24, 40

Yehuda, R. 32
Yontef, G.M. 48, 54, 55
Young, H. 59

Zana, K. 4, 89, 104, 116, 122

For Product Safety Concerns and Information please contact our EU
representative GPSR@taylorandfrancis.com
Taylor & Francis Verlag GmbH, Kaufingerstraße 24, 80331 München, Germany